Praise for *Johns Hopkins Nursing Evidence-Based Practice: Model and Guidelines, Third Edition*

"Part of the challenge of teaching the EBP process is how to keep it simple so frontline staff can understand the process and stop seeing it as so complex that only nurses pursuing graduate studies can comprehend. That is where this book comes in handy. The Johns Hopkins Nursing Evidence-Based Practice PET (Practice question, Evidence, and Translation) process is explained in an understandable, guiding manner from beginning to end. In addition to helping one be organized, the tools are an integral part of further understanding the EBP components. The exemplars make EBP 'doable' and thus relatable. It is impressive that cited EBP projects were implemented by a single nurse or team of nurses, ranging from frontline staff to multidisciplinary teams, and including partnering physicians. The book also covers how to overcome barriers to EBP and how to sustain change achieved from implementing the process. This book gives nurses the knowledge and power to disseminate EBP, and it is not far-fetched to expect EBP to be a nursing habit."

–Ruth Bala-Kerr, MSN, RN, CNS, CPHQ, NE-BC
Director, Clinical Professional Development
Harbor-UCLA Medical Center

"As a clinical nurse leader and EBP champion, I absolutely love the *Johns Hopkins Nursing Evidence-Based Practice: Model and Guidelines* book; it is my all-time favorite resource book on the subject. I had the opportunity to attend a Johns Hopkins EBP boot camp, and while reading this book, I felt as though I was having that amazing experience again! This book is easy to read and a great tool for nurses on any level of proficiency. I recommend it as a practical way to integrate EBP into any practice environment."

–Kimberly M. Barnes, MSN, RN, CNL
Clinical Nurse Leader, Patient Care Services

"In 2006, our organization chose to adopt the Johns Hopkins Nursing Evidence-Based Practice Model because of its ease of use and its tools for nurses with diverse educational backgrounds. With each new edition, the authors improve the quality and function of this model. This third edition provides further depth and clarification with the addition of a new chapter, 'Lessons From Practice: Using the JHNEBP Tools,' and translation tools that provide clear, concise instruction. We will continue to use this book as a resource for our nurses and allied health professionals in developing their knowledge and skills in identification and translation of evidence into daily clinical and administrative decision-making."

–Barbara L. Buchko, DNP, RNC-MNN
Director of Evidence-Based Practice and Nursing Research
WellSpan Health

"In early 2000, The Johns Hopkins Hospital (JHH) Post Anesthesia Care Unit (PACU) was very fortunate to be the pilot site for the Johns Hopkins Nursing Evidence-Based Practice Model. PACU nurses from inpatient and ambulatory settings were invited to participate. There was a sense of staff reluctance and lack of appreciation for what their involvement meant. Seeing the nurses' active engagement in the pilot and outcome was every nurse manager's dream. Using evidence in making decisions became a reality. *Johns Hopkins Nursing Evidence-Based Practice: Model and Guidelines, Third Edition,* captures the essence of nursing excellence in practice. This book illustrates the barriers in today's nursing practice in developing critical thinking and competence; it provides the structure, process, tools, and measurement of outcomes for proficiency levels ranging from nursing students to leaders and for every setting. I am most grateful to Johns Hopkins for its nursing leadership in the culture of inquiry."

–Dina A. Krenzischek, PhD, RN, CPAN, CFRE, FAAN
Director of Professional Practice
Mercy Medical Center

"*Johns Hopkins Nursing Evidence-Based Practice: Model and Guidelines* is very practical, with clarity about how to determine evidence levels and additional factors that influence practice. The new model is active and interrelating. Support materials available to end users are reasonably priced, practical, and helpful to bedside nurses who conduct evidence-based practice projects. We use these materials for EBP improvement, EBP internships, and nurse residency. Model elements are easy to understand and explain. The detailed, stepwise progression from forming a team and clinical question to disseminating findings guides a comprehensive and systematic approach to EBP. The focus on translation of best evidence into practice addresses one of the most challenging and critical phases of EBP. Our Organizational Nursing Research Council adopted the JHNEBP Model and has been using the support materials for almost 10 years. The exemplars are helpful in supporting learning. Our hospital purchased the ebook, and we look forward to updating to the third edition."

–Debra Haas Stavarski, PhD, MS, RN
Director of Nursing Research
Reading Hospital, Reading Health System

Johns Hopkins Nursing
Evidence-Based Practice:
Model and Guidelines
Third Edition

Deborah Dang, PhD, RN, NEA-BC
Sandra L. Dearholt, MS, RN, NEA-BC

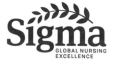

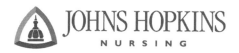

The Sigma Theta Tau International Honor Society of Nursing (Sigma) is a nonprofit organization whose mission is advancing world health and celebrating nursing excellence in scholarship, leadership, and service. Founded in 1922, Sigma has more than 135,000 active members in over 90 countries and territories. Members include practicing nurses, instructors, researchers, policymakers, entrepreneurs, and others. Sigma's more than 530 chapters are located at more than 700 institutions of higher education throughout Armenia, Australia, Botswana, Brazil, Canada, Colombia, England, Ghana, Hong Kong, Japan, Jordan, Kenya, Lebanon, Malawi, Mexico, the Netherlands, Pakistan, Philippines, Portugal, Singapore, South Africa, South Korea, Swaziland, Sweden, Taiwan, Tanzania, Thailand, the United States, and Wales. Learn more at www.sigmanursing.org.

Sigma Nursing
550 West North Street
Indianapolis, IN, USA 46202

To order additional books, buy in bulk, or order for corporate use, contact Sigma Marketplace at 888.654.4968 (US and Canada) or +1.317.634.8171 (outside US and Canada).

To request a review copy for course adoption, email solutions@sigmamarketplace.org or call 888.654.4968 (US and Canada) or +1.317.634.8171 (outside US and Canada).

To request author information, or for speaker or other media requests, contact Sigma Marketing at 888.634.7575 (US and Canada) or +1.317.634.8171 (outside US and Canada).

ISBN:	9781940446974
EPUB ISBN:	9781940446981
PDF ISBN:	9781940446998
MOBI ISBN:	9781945157004

Library of Congress Cataloging-in-Publication Data

Names: Dang, Deborah, editor. | Dearholt, Sandra, editor. | Sigma Theta Tau International. | Johns Hopkins University. School of Nursing.
Title: Johns Hopkins nursing evidence-based practice : model & guidelines / [edited by] Deborah Dang, Sandra L. Dearholt.
Other titles: Johns Hopkins nursing evidence-based practice (Dearholt). | Nursing evidence-based practice
Description: Third edition. | Indianapolis, IN : Sigma Theta Tau International, [2018] | Sandra Dearholt's name appears first on the previous edition. | Includes bibliographical references and index.
Identifiers: LCCN 2017039003 (print) | LCCN 2017039732 (ebook) | ISBN 9781940446981 (Epub) | ISBN 9781940446998 (Pdf) | ISBN 9781945157004 (Mobi) | ISBN 9781940446974 (print : alk. paper) | ISBN 9781945157004 (mobi)
Subjects: | MESH: Evidence-Based Nursing | Models, Nursing | Evidence-Based Nursing | Models, Nursing
Classification: LCC RT42 (ebook) | LCC RT42 (print) | NLM WY 100.7 | DDC 610.73--dc23
LC record available at https://lccn.loc.gov/2017039003

Third Printing, 2019

Publisher: Dustin Sullivan
Acquisitions Editor: Emily Hatch
Editorial Coordinator: Paula Jeffers
Cover Designer: Rebecca Batchelor
Interior Design/Page Layout: Rebecca Batchelor

Principal Book Editor: Carla Hall
Development and Project Editor: Kevin Kent
Copy Editor: Becky Whitney
Proofreader: Gill Editorial Services
Indexer: Joy Dean Lee

DEDICATION

This book is dedicated to those nurses everywhere—consummate professionals in whatever setting they practice—who are committed to excellence in patient care based on best available evidence.

ACKNOWLEDGMENTS

We would like to acknowledge the insight and expertise of the authors of the first edition (2007) of *Johns Hopkins Nursing Evidence-Based Practice: Model and Guidelines*: **Robin P. Newhouse**, PhD, RN, NEA-BC, FAAN; **Sandra L. Dearholt, MS, RN, NEA-BC**; Stephanie S. Poe, DNP, RN; **Linda C. Pugh**, PhD, RNC, CNE, FAAN; and **Kathleen M. White**, PhD, RN, NEA-BC, FAAN.

The foundational work of these experts transformed evidence-based practice into a process that promotes autonomy and provides frontline nurses with the competencies and tools to apply the best evidence to improve patient care. The profession as a whole is indebted to them.

ABOUT THE EDITORS

Deborah Dang, PhD, RN, NEA-BC

Deborah Dang is the director of nursing practice, education and research at The Johns Hopkins Hospital. In her current position, she developed the strategic vision for evidence-based practice (EBP) at The Johns Hopkins Hospital, and built an infrastructure that has enabled the transformation to practice based on evidence. Throughout her tenure she led and championed nursing professional practice. Cultivating its growth from the initial model development to final implementation, she co-created, with clinical nurses and nurse leaders, the components of The Johns Hopkins Hospital Professional Practice Model: the philosophy of nursing, the clinical advancement program, professional development for frontline leaders and staff, salaried compensation, shared governance, and evidence-based practice, thus building an infrastructure to continually advance nursing excellence. As a health services researcher, her funded studies focus on disruptive behavior, positive psychology, and mindful leadership. Dang has published, consulted, and presented nationally and internationally on the subject of EBP. She also holds a joint appointment with The Johns Hopkins University School of Nursing.

Sandra L. Dearholt, MS, RN, NEA-BC

Sandra L. Dearholt is assistant director of nursing for the Departments of Neurosciences and Psychiatry Nursing at The Johns Hopkins Hospital. Dearholt has written numerous articles on EBP and has extensive experience in the development and delivery of EBP educational programs. Her areas of interest focus on strategies for incorporating EBP into practice at the bedside, the development of professional practice standards, and fostering service excellence. She is a co-author of the first edition of *Johns Hopkins Nursing Evidence-Based Practice: Model and Guidelines* and a contributing author to *Johns Hopkins Nursing Evidence-Based Practice: Implementation and Translation*.

ABOUT THE CONTRIBUTING AUTHORS

Chapter 1: Evidence-Based Practice: Context, Concerns, and Challenges

Linda C. Pugh, PhD, RN, RNC, FAAN

Linda Pugh is a professor of nursing at the University of North Carolina Wilmington and the past director of evidence-based practice/nursing research at the York Hospital of Pennsylvania. Pugh co-authored the first edition of *Johns Hopkins Nursing Evidence-Based Practice: Model and Guidelines.* As a certified obstetric nurse, she has provided care for childbearing women for over 35 years and has taught nursing at the baccalaureate, masters, and doctoral levels. She has been the recipient of numerous grants to support her research on improving breastfeeding outcomes particularly with low-income women. Pugh has published and presented her work internationally and nationally.

Chapter 2: Critical Thinking and Evidence-Based Practice

Stephanie S. Poe, DNP, RN, RN-BC

Stephanie S. Poe is senior director of nursing quality and informatics at The Johns Hopkins Hospital and the chief nursing information officer for The Johns Hopkins Hospital and Health System. Poe is widely published and is considered an expert in patient safety, quality, and clinical informatics. She is one of the original developers of the Johns Hopkins Nursing Evidence-Based Practice Model and Guidelines and the Johns Hopkins Fall Risk Assessment Tool, both of which have been widely used nationally and internationally. She served as an editor of the *Johns Hopkins Nursing Evidence-Based Practice: Implementation and Translation* and *Measuring Patient Safety* books. Her research areas of interest are patient portals, building capacity for informatics, fall risk assessment, and medication reconciliation.

Sharon Dudley Brown, PhD, CRNP

Sharon Dudley-Brown currently is an assistant professor at Johns Hopkins University, in the Schools of Nursing & Medicine, Baltimore, Maryland. She is also the co-director of the Nurse Practitioner Fellowship Program in Gastro-enterology & Hepatology at Johns Hopkins. She sees patients and conducts research on patients with inflammatory bowel disease. Dudley-Brown has held several academic appointments, both nationally and internationally, and has worked as a nurse practitioner at several institutions over the past 25 years. She has published several peer-reviewed papers and abstracts in the fields of nursing, inflammatory bowel disease, and ulcerative colitis, and she is currently a member of several editorial boards, including *Gastroenterology Nursing Journal*, where she is the online editor. She is a co-editor of a textbook on translation in evidence-based practice, *Translation of Evidence into Nursing and Health Care* published by Springer, just out in a second edition. In addition, Dudley-Brown is a member of many professional societies, including the Society of Gastrointestinal Nurses and Associates (SGNA), American Academy of Nurse Practitioners (AANP), the American Gastroenterological Association (AGA), and the American College of Gastroenterology (ACG). Additionally, she is an active member of the Crohn's and Colitis Foundation of America (CCFA), serving on the National Nursing Initiatives Committee, as well as on her local Medical Advisory Committee.

Sue C. Verrillo, DNP, RN, CRRN

Sue C. Verrillo is the nurse manager of the Ortho/Ortho-Spine/Trauma Unit at The Johns Hopkins Hospital. Verrillo is a member of The Johns Hopkins Hospital EBP Steering Committee and was a guest author for the second edition of *Johns Hopkins Nursing Evidence-Based Practice: Implementation and Translation*. As a certified rehabilitation nurse, she has provided leadership for nursing staff excellence, for the expansion of the unit, and for maintaining the unit's national certification. She has conducted quality improvement outcome studies on the orthopedic unit on the relationship of inpatient continuous postoperative vital sign monitoring and failure to rescue. She has published and presented her work nationally and internationally.

Chapter 3: The Johns Hopkins Nursing Evidence-Based Practice Model and Process Overview

Sandra L. Dearholt, MS, RN, NEA-BC

See Sandra L. Dearholt's bio earlier.

Sharon H. Allan, DNP, RN, ACNS-BC, CCRC

Sharon Allan is a clinical nurse specialist at The Johns Hopkins Hospital. She is chair of Nursing Standards of Care Committee, overseeing evidence-based policy and protocol development and review. She has published, presented, and consulted nationally on clinical research studies, quality improvement, and evidence-based practice projects. Her funded studies focused on heart/lung transplant, best practices in a cardiac surgery ICU, and clinical alarm management. Allan is a member of NACNS, STTI, AACN, AAMI, and the ANA.

Chapter 4: The Practice Question

Robin P. Newhouse, PhD, RN, NEA-BC, FAAN

Robin Newhouse is distinguished professor and dean of the Indiana University School of Nursing. Her research focuses on health system interventions to improve care processes and patient outcomes. She has published extensively on health services improvement interventions, acute care quality issues, and evidence-based practice. Newhouse co-authored the first edition of the *Johns Hopkins Nursing Evidence-Based Practice: Model and Guidelines*. Newhouse is a member of the American Nurses Credentialing Center's Research Council, past chair of the Research and Scholarship Advisory Council for Sigma Theta Tau International Honor Society of Nursing, and serves on the Academy Health Board and the Patient Centered Outcomes Research Institute Methodology Committee. She was inducted into the Sigma Theta Tau International Honor Society of Nursing Nurse Researcher Hall of Fame and received the American Nurses Credentialing Center President's Award in 2015.

Chapter 5: Searching for Evidence

Stella Seal, MLS

Stella Seal is the associate director for hospital, health system, and community services at the Welch Medical Library, Johns Hopkins Medical Institutions. She has more than 20 years of experience providing information services to the faculty, students, and staff of The Johns Hopkins School of Nursing. Seal has presented numerous instructional sessions on all aspects of database searching and research tools, in addition to her collaborations on grant proposals and systematic reviews.

Christina L. Wissinger, PhD

Christina L. Wissinger is a tenure track faculty member with the Pennsylvania State University Libraries. In addition to her PhD, she holds a master's degree in library and information science. She has worked in several academic health sciences libraries, including Johns Hopkins, collaborating with nurses, allied health professionals, clinicians, and biomedical researchers. Wissinger consults on grant-funded research projects and systematic reviews, and conducts CE sessions. Her scholarship focuses on literacy, privacy, informed consent, health communications, and medical humanities.

Elizabeth Scala, MSN/MBA, RN

Elizabeth Scala is the research program coordinator at The Johns Hopkins Hospital. In addition to assisting with the Nursing Research Program, Elizabeth supports clinical nurses to develop enhanced knowledge and skills in nursing research.

Chapter 6: Evidence Appraisal: Research

Linda Costa, PhD, RN, NEA-BC

Linda Costa is an assistant professor at the University of Maryland School of Nursing in the Department of Organizational Systems and Adult Health. She has presented and consulted nationally and internationally on the topic of evidence-based practice and leadership. As a health services researcher, her funded studies focus on medication management, nurse's contribution to discharge transitions, and post-discharge outcomes. She teaches practice leadership within complex adaptive healthcare systems, translating evidence to practice and methods for research and evidence-based practice.

Jennifer Day, PhD, RN

Jennifer Day is the director of nursing research at the University of Maryland Medical Center, Baltimore and consulting associate at Duke University School of Nursing. Day mentors clinical nurses in both evidence-based practice and nursing research. Her research focus is on older adults and family caregivers; her work on compassion fatigue has received NIH funding. She has presented and published on these topics, in addition to how to engage clinical nurses in nursing research and building PhD and DNP-prepared nurse partnerships for improved patient outcomes.

Chapter 7: Evidence Appraisal: Nonresearch

Hayley D. Mark, PhD, MPH, RN, FAAN

Hayley D. Mark is professor and chair in the Department of Nursing at Towson University in Towson, Maryland. Mark's research expertise is in sexually transmitted infections and sexual health, and she is widely published on these topics. Mark has also presented nationally and internationally on the topic of evidence-based practice in nursing. She has taught research methods to undergraduate and graduate nursing students for over 15 years.

Hyunjeong Park, PhD, MPH, MSN, RN

Hyunjeong Park is an assistant professor in the Department of Nursing at Towson University. She has taught research methods to nursing students and has expertise in facilitating evidence-based projects that expand collaboration between students and diverse populations in community health nursing. Park has also presented and published evidence-based research internationally.

Chapter 8: Translation

Kathleen White, PhD, RN, NEA-BC, FAAN

Kathleen White is a professor at The Johns Hopkins University School of Nursing. White has authored multiple publications on the Johns Hopkins Nursing EBP model and consults and presents on this subject. White co-authored the first edition of *Johns Hopkins Nursing Evidence-Based Practice: Model and Guidelines* and co-edited *Johns Hopkins Nursing Evidence-Based Practice: Implementation and Translation.*

Robin P. Newhouse, PhD, RN, NEA-BC, FAAN

See Robin P. Newhouse's bio earlier.

Chapter 9: Creating a Supportive EBP Environment

Kathleen White, PhD, RN, NEA-BC, FAAN

See Kathleen White's bio earlier.

Deborah Dang, PhD, RN, NEA-BC

See Deborah Dang's bio earlier.

Chapter 10: Exemplars

Kim Bissett, MSN/MBA, RN

Kim Bissett is a nurse educator and EBP specialist at the Institute for Johns Hopkins Nursing. She was the inaugural Evidence-Based Practice Coordinator at The Johns Hopkins Hospital, following two years of serving as the EBP fellow. She currently chairs the EBP Steering Committee and has led and participated in numerous EBP projects. Bissett has presented on the topic of evidence-based nursing practice both nationally and internationally.

Deborah Dang, PhD, RN, NEA-BC

See Deborah Dang's bio earlier.

Sandra L. Dearholt, MS, RN, NEA-BC

See Sandra L. Dearholt's bio earlier.

Those contributing exemplars to the chapter were as follows:

Establishing the Access in Minutes Team in the Adult Emergency Department

Madeleine Whalen, MSN/MPH, RN, CEN

Diana-Lyn Baptiste, DNP, RN

Barbara Maliszewski, MS, RN

The Johns Hopkins Hospital Baltimore, MD, USA

Drawing aPTT Samples from Central Lines While Heparin Is Concurrently Infusing

Daniel Hare, BSN, RN, PCCN

Margaret Witman, RN, PCCN

Candice Penaranda, BSN, RN

Jennifer Mayo, BSN, RN

Christina Ewing, BSN, RN

Barbara Palm, RN

Nicole Bahadursingh, RN

Ashley Ewald, RN

Capucine Dingle, RN

Heidi Mock, RN

Tania Fletcher, BSN, RN

Karen Keim, MSN, RN

Heidi Chroszielewski, MSN, RN-BC, PCCN

Mercy Medical Center Baltimore, MD, USA

Initiating Purposeful Hourly Rounding on an Inpatient Oncology Unit to Improve Patient Safety and Satisfaction

Laurie Bryant, MSN, RN, OCN, ACNS-BC

Irina Rifkind, MSN, RN

Sarah McCarthy, BSN, RN

The Johns Hopkins Hospital Baltimore, MD, USA

The Effectiveness of Sennosides to Decrease Constipation Post Uterine Artery Embolization (UAE)

> Dana Triplett, BSN, RN, CCRN
>
> Deborah Phillips, RN, CRN
>
> Suzanne Stiffler, BSN, RN, RN-BC
>
> Jane Hauhn, RN, CCRN
>
> Theresa Neskow-Logan, RN
>
> Andrea Staiti, BSN, RN
>
> Brad Cogan, MD
>
> Robert Liddell, MD
>
> David Sill, MD
>
> Mercy Medical Center
>
> Baltimore, MD, USA

Wipe Out CAUTI: Implementing Nonbasin Bathing to Reduce CAUTIs

> Abigail C. Strouse, DNP, RN, ACNS-BC, NEA-BC, CBN
>
> WellSpan Health York Hospital York, PA, USA

Chapter 11: Lessons from Practice: Using the JHNEBP Tools

Kim Bissett, MSN, MBA, RN

> See Kim Bissett's bio earlier.

Table of Contents

Foreword

I am thrilled to present the third edition of *Johns Hopkins Nursing Evidence-Based Practice: Model and Guidelines*. This new edition reaffirms the original mission of the Johns Hopkins Nursing Evidence-Based Practice (JHNEBP) model: "Support the safety of our patients, the development of our profession, and the education of our students." Patient outcomes and clinician-peer feedback have contributed greatly to this edition that we hope supports nursing as the United States' most trusted profession.

In the late 1990s, U.S. experts drew all of our attention to the alarming number of medical mistakes related to poor communication and variation in care standards through the groundbreaking report, *To Err Is Human* (Institute of Medicine, 2000). The Institute of Medicine's (IOM) work catapulted nursing's transition from focusing solely on applying new knowledge to connecting that knowledge to patient outcomes with the goal of improving healthcare quality. Over the past decade, nursing has been called to lead interprofessional care teams within an expectant healthcare system. These expectations have resulted in the development of best practices at all levels of nursing that require evidence-based competencies.

Johns Hopkins nursing has a well-earned reputation for questioning traditional practice decisions, which provides a rich environment for the development of evidence-based guidelines. In this third edition, the revised JHNEBP model incorporates this spirit of inquiry promoting the scientific examination of practice questions and the appraisal of evidence. The translation of the highest quality of evidence is used to inform both learning and nursing practice. In collaboration with patients, families, and caregivers, nurses impact improvements in healthcare quality, safety, equity, and values as outlined in the Institute of Medicine Report: *The Future of Nursing* (2011).

This third edition of the JHNEBP model and guidelines has been revised to include learning from 10 years of use in practice and feedback provided by numerous clinicians, educators, and students from around the world. The authors continue to meet the demands posited by our patients, caregivers, and inquisitive and dynamic nursing workforce to apply the best evidence to our practices, including newer approaches in population health and the provision of value-based care.

I am proud to endorse this continued commitment to evidence-based practice and inquiry that supports nurses in reducing care variation in the pursuit of patient safety and quality. These efforts contribute to developing the competencies of nurses all over the globe.

–Deborah Baker, DNP

References

Institute of Medicine. (2000). *To err is human*. Washington D.C.: The National Academies Press.

Institute of Medicine. (2011). *The future of nursing: Leading change, advancing health*. Washington D.C.: The National Academies Press.

Introduction

Johns Hopkins Nursing Evidence-Based Practice: Model and Guidelines (JH-NEBP) is steadfastly dedicated to the advancement of evidence-based practice (EBP) and to frontline nurses who strive daily to improve patient care outcomes through the translation of evidence into practice. Revisions to the third edition have been informed by over a decade of experience using the model and from the genuine and generous feedback received by clinicians and nursing students across the country as they apply the process in real-life settings. As we progress on our journey to enhance the JHNEBP model and guidelines to facilitate the implementation of EBP, we are grateful to those nurses who have taken the time to provide feedback to improve the clarity and usability of the model in a variety of clinical and academic settings. In this third edition, we are excited to be able to share these changes.

The new edition lays the foundation for understanding the importance of implementing EBP in a transformed healthcare environment, emphasizing the necessity for continuous quality improvement and cost effectiveness. The JH-NEBP model has been reconceptualized to capture the need for organizations to cultivate both a spirit of inquiry and an environment of learning that encourages questioning, seeking best evidence and the implementation of innovative improvements. The third edition also highlights EBP as a core competency for all healthcare professionals. The Affordable Care Act has opened the doors for funding related to the advancement of interprofessional collaboration and teamwork particularly when addressing complex patient care issues such as those often tackled by EBP teams. Additionally, the tools used to guide the EBP process have been updated, and a number of new tools (Stakeholder Analysis, Action Planning, and Dissemination) have been added. The third edition also includes a new chapter on important tips for using the EBP tools.

The third edition continues to carry on the tradition first established by M. Adelaide Nutting, Assistant Superintendent of nurses at The Johns Hopkins

Hospital, Principal of The Johns Hopkins School of Nursing, and pioneer in the development of nursing education:

> *We need to realize and affirm a view that "medicine" is one of the most difficult of arts. Compassion may provide the motive but knowledge is our only working power.... Surely we will not be satisfied with merely perpetuating methods and traditions; surely we should be more and more involved with creating them.*

Evidence-Based Practice Background

Evidence-Based Practice: Context, Concerns, and Challenges

Evidence-based practice (EBP) is one of the core competencies for all healthcare providers (Institute of Medicine [IOM], 2003). Nurses are part of the interprofessional team and have a significant influence on healthcare decisions and improving quality and safety of care. Beyond an expectation for professional practice, EBP provides a major opportunity for nurses to improve practice and add value to the patient experience. The Institute leaders also advocated (IOM, 2010) that nurses become full partners in the redesign of healthcare systems to improve the quality of care. This report suggested the need for a strong foundation in *evidence-based* care to accomplish this goal. Further, Dr. Patricia A. Grady, director of the National Institute for Nursing Research, stated that, "Nurse scientists are well positioned to take leadership roles and serve as catalysts" in the field of translational science—that is, translating research into everyday practice (Grady, 2010, p. 166). Discovery of new knowledge alone does not have an impact unless it is translated into practice. The ability to base the practice of nursing on strong evidence is an essential competency for contemporary nursing practice. Perhaps the strongest support for addressing a healthcare system dedicated to providing the best care with the best outcomes was proposed by the Quality and Safety Education for Nurses (QSEN) project, funded by the Robert Wood Johnson Foundation. QSEN has identified core competencies for all registered nurses (QSEN, 2016). Nurses need the knowledge, skills, and attitude in these core competencies: patient-centered care, teamwork and collaboration, EBP, quality improvement, safety, and informatics. Using the best evidence to provide healthcare is required in order to realize healthcare improvements and cost savings. The objectives for this chapter are to:

- Define EBP
- Describe the evolution of EBP in the nursing profession
- Discuss EBP in relation to outcomes and accountability
- Highlight nursing's role in EBP

EBP: A Definition

EBP is a problem-solving approach to clinical decision-making within a healthcare organization. EBP integrates the best available scientific evidence with the best available experiential (patient and practitioner) evidence. EBP considers internal and external influences on practice and encourages critical thinking in the judicious application of such evidence to the care of individual patients, a patient population, or a system (Dearholt & Dang, 2012). EBP uses current research and nonresearch evidence to produce high-quality healthcare. The challenge for healthcare providers is to use such evidence to implement the best interventions to improve patient outcomes.

EBP supports and informs clinical, administrative, and educational decision-making. Combining research, organizational experience (including quality improvement and financial data), clinical expertise, expert opinion, and patient preferences ensures clinical decisions are based on all available evidence. EBP enhances *efficacy* (the ability to reach a desired result); *efficiency* (the achievement of a desired result with minimum expense, time, and effort); and *effectiveness* (the ability to produce a desired result). Additionally, EBP weighs risk, benefit, and cost against a backdrop of patient preferences. This evidence-based decision-making encourages healthcare providers to question practice and determine which interventions are ready to be implemented in clinical practice. EBP can lead to optimal outcomes, equivalent care at lower cost and in less time, improved patient satisfaction, and higher health-related quality of life.

Differentiating Quality Improvement, Research, and EBP

Nurses are often perplexed about differences between the three forms of inquiry: quality improvement (QI), research, and EBP. Although QI, research, and EBP use distinctly different processes, commonalities among these three concepts include teamwork, critical thinking, and a commitment to improve care. The methods used and outcomes sought are different for each type of inquiry (see Table 1.1).

Table 1.1   Differentiating Three Forms of Nursing Inquiry

	Quality Improvement	Research	EBP
Starting point	Gap in performance for practice, process, or system	Gap in knowledge evidence	Gap in knowledge of best available evidence
Method used	Plan-Do-Study-Act (PDSA)	Scientific process	Practice Question, Evidence, Translation (PET)
Outcome	Produces evidence for application at local level (unit, department, organization)	Generates new knowledge for broad application	Synthesizes best evidence for adoption in practice

Quality improvement is a process to improve healthcare services, systems, and processes at the local level (i.e., unit, department, organization) with the intent to improve outcomes (U.S. Department of Health and Human Services, 2016). QI generally includes a method of measuring a particular outcome, making changes to improve practice, and monitoring performance on an ongoing basis. QI may uncover a practice problem that initiates an EBP project. Some examples of QI initiatives are decreasing catheter-associated urinary tract infections, decreasing wait times in the emergency department, decreasing falls among patients, decreasing surgical site infections, improving patient satisfaction, improving pneumococcal and influenza immunization rates, and decreasing restraint use.

Research is a systematic investigation (quantitative, qualitative, or mixed methods) designed to develop, uncover, create, or contribute to new knowledge that can be generalized for broader application (U.S. Department of Health and Human Services, 2009, 45 CFR 46.102[d]). It is often undertaken when no evidence is found during an EBP project. Research involves approval by an institutional review board. Some examples of research are investigating pain in the ventilated patient; communication between caregivers, family, and patient at the end of life; and post-stroke memory function.

An EBP project is undertaken when clinicians have a particular concern or question about their practice. The EBP process includes identifying a practice problem and EBP question, locating the best available evidence, appraising the level and quality of evidence, and synthesizing findings leading to translation of evidence into practice. One example is performing mouth care every four hours on ventilated patients because the evidence shows that it helps decrease the incidence of ventilator-associated pneumonia and mortality, cost, and length of stay. A second example is using warm-water compresses to manage nipple pain in breastfeeding mothers.

While these three forms of inquiry are distinct, they are linked when determining a course of action based on the nature of the question or problem raised by nurses. As depicted in Figure 1.1, a frontline nurse raised the issue of increased infection rates in orthopedic patients with traction pins. Initially, efforts to decrease rates began as a QI project. On studying the current practice using the PDSA method, the team discovered that there was variation in pin care among the nurses. The unit staff then undertook an EBP project to find the best available evidence on pin care. Finding no evidence in their search, they initiated a research study to generate new knowledge on the most effective pin care cleaning protocol for minimizing infection.

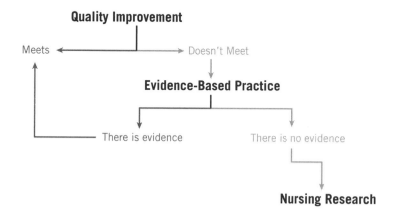

Figure 1.1   Choosing a form of inquiry for practice problems.

The History

EBP is not conceptually new. As with any applied science, the terms associated with EBP changed as the science evolved. As early as 1972, Archibald L. Cochrane, a British medical researcher, criticized the health profession for administering treatments not supported by evidence (Cochrane, 1972). By the 1980s, the term *evidence-based medicine* was being used at McMaster University Medical School in Canada. Positive reception given to systematic reviews of care during pregnancy and childbirth prompted the British National Health Service in 1992 to approve funding for "a Cochrane Centre" to facilitate the preparation of systematic reviews of randomized controlled trials of healthcare, eventually leading to the establishment of the Cochrane Collaboration in 1993 (The Cochrane Collaboration, 2016). Cochrane provides systematic reviews about the effectiveness of healthcare and sound scientific evidence for providing effective treatment regimes.

Research utilization was the initial effort to promote the translation of research into practice. The use of tradition and ritual was a strong basis for care by many nurses. In an effort to use research in clinical practice, the Western Interstate Commission for Higher Education (WICHE) initiated the first major nurse-based EBP project (Krueger, 1978). Research, a relatively new professional discipline for nurses, was just beginning to develop; nurses were interested in conducting research useful to clinicians. Nursing science targeted the study of nurses at this time rather than examining the impact of clinical interventions used in practice.

Another early attempt at using research in practice was the Conduct and Utilization of Research in Nursing Project (CURN) (Horsley, Crane, & Bingle, 1978). Ten areas were identified as having adequate evidence to use in practice (Horsley, Crane, Crabtree, & Wood, 1983):

- Structured preoperative teaching
- Reducing diarrhea in tube-fed patients
- Preoperative sensory preparation to promote recovery
- Prevention of decubitus ulcers
- Intravenous cannula change
- Closed urinary drainage systems
- Distress reduction through sensory preparation
- Mutual goal setting in patient care
- Clean intermittent catheterization
- Deliberate nursing interventions to reduce pain

These efforts were the beginning of using research in practice. EBP is more than research utilization as science; experience, patient preference, and internal organizational data are all used to improve patient outcomes. Building on these early efforts, EBP has developed to include increasingly sophisticated analytical techniques; improved presentation and dissemination of information; growing knowledge of how to implement findings while effectively considering patient preferences, costs, and policy issues; and a better understanding of how to measure effect and use feedback to promote ongoing improvement.

EBP and Outcomes

Healthcare providers, by nature, have always been interested in the outcomes and results of patient care. Traditionally, such results have been characterized in terms of morbidity and mortality. Recently, however, the focus has broadened to include *clinical outcomes* (e.g., hospital-acquired infection, falls, pressure ulcers), *functional outcomes* (e.g., performance of daily activities), *quality-of-life outcomes* (e.g., physical and mental health), and *economic outcomes* (e.g., direct, indirect, and intangible costs). EBP is an explicit process by which clinicians conduct critical evidence reviews and examine the link between healthcare practices and outcomes to inform decisions and improve the quality of care and patient safety.

EBP and Accountability

Nowhere is accountability a more sensitive topic than in healthcare. Knowing that patient outcomes are linked to evidence-based interventions is critical for promoting quality patient care. It is also mandated by professional and regulatory organizations and third-party payers, and is expected by patients and families. Medical error is thought to be a leading cause of death among hospitalized patients (Makary & Daniel, 2016). Public expectations that healthcare investments lead to high-quality results most likely will not diminish in the near future. In today's environment, quality and cost concerns drive healthcare. Consumers expect professionals to deliver the best evidence-based care with the least amount of risk.

Much of the information available suggests that consumers are not consistently receiving appropriate care (IOM, 2001). Nurses and other healthcare professionals operate within an age of accountability (Leonenko & Drach-Zahavy, 2016); this accountability has become a focal point for healthcare (Pronovost, 2010). It is within this environment that nurses, physicians, public health scientists, and others explore what works and does not, and it is within this context that nurses and other healthcare providers continue the journey to bridge research and practice.

Governments and society challenge healthcare providers to base their practices on current, validated interventions. In 2011, the director of the National Institutes of Health, Dr. Francis S. Collins, proposed the National Center for Advancing Translational Sciences, whose aim it is to accelerate the translation of scientific discoveries into practice. The director of this exciting center, Dr. Christopher Austin, announced new funding streams to strengthen translational science and the movement of discovery concerning disease and patient outcomes into everyday practice (Austin, 2016). Nursing has responded to the groundswell of information by educating nurses at every level to be competent practitioners of EBP and to close the gap between research and practice (Melnyk, Gallagher-Ford, Long, & Fineout-Overholt, 2014).

EBP provides a systematic approach to decision-making that leads to best practices and demonstrates nurse accountability for the care they provide. When the strongest available evidence is considered, the odds of doing the right thing at the right time for the right patient are improved. Given the complexity of linking research and clinical practice, EBP provides the most useful framework to translate evidence into practice.

Knowing and Using Evidence

In healthcare, unfortunately, more is known than is practiced. The process of incorporating new knowledge into clinical practice is often considerably delayed. Collins (2011) reports that it takes, on average, 13 years to approve new drugs. The average time for the uptake of research into actual practice is 17 years (Hanney et al., 2015). New knowledge has grown exponentially. Early in the 20th century, professional nurses had but a few, hard-to-access journals available to them. Today, MEDLINE indexes 5,600 journals (National Library of Medicine, 2016) with more than 26 million references. The Cumulative Index to Nursing and Allied Health Literature (CINAHL) indexes more than 3,100 journals and includes more than 3.4 million records (Ebsco Publishing, 2016). Accessibility of information on the Web also has increased consumer expectation of participating in treatment decisions. Patients with chronic health problems have accumulated considerable expertise in self-management, increasing the pressure for providers to be up-to-date with the best evidence for care.

Despite this knowledge explosion, healthcare clinicians can experience a decline in knowledge of best care practices that relates to the amount of information available and the limited time to digest it. Estabrooks (1998) reported that knowledge of best care practices negatively correlated with year of graduation—that is, knowledge of best care practices declined as the number of years since graduation increased. EBP is one of the best strategies to enable nurses to stay abreast of new practices and technology amid this continuing information explosion.

Nursing's Role in EBP

EBP encompasses multiple sources of knowledge, clinical expertise, and patient preference. Because of their unique position and expertise at the bedside, nurses often play a pivotal role in generating questions about patient care and safety. This, along with the fact that practice questions and concerns often cross disciplines, makes it critical to enlist an interprofessional team and to include patient and family input as part of the process. Thus, nurses need to develop the necessary knowledge and skills to not only participate in an EBP process but also serve as leaders of interdisciplinary EBP teams seeking best practices to improve patient care. Nurses and nursing leaders also play a central role in modeling and promoting a culture that supports the use of collaborative EBP within the organization and in ensuring that the necessary resources (e.g., time, education, equipment, mentors, and library support) are in place to facilitate and sustain the process. Ways to be current include: reading widely and critically, attending professional conferences, expecting evidence that a procedure is effective, becoming involved in a journal club, and participating in EBP projects. The Johns Hopkins Nursing EBP model is an effective and efficient method to begin the EBP process. The model has been used in many institutions and has been embraced by front-line nurses. The tools developed as part of the model enable the nurse to use a step-by-step process for successfully completing an EBP project.

Summary

This chapter defines EBP and discusses the evolution that led to the critical need for practice based on evidence to guide decision-making. EBP creates a culture of critical thinking and ongoing learning and is the foundation for an environment in which evidence supports clinical, administrative, and educational decisions. EBP supports rational decision-making, reducing inappropriate variation in practice, and making it easier for nurses to do their job.

Numbering more than 3 million and practicing in all healthcare settings, nurses make up the largest number of health professionals. Every patient is likely to receive nursing care; therefore, nurses are in a position to influence the type, quality, and cost of care provided to patients. For nursing, the framework for decision-making has traditionally been the nursing process. Understood in this framework is the use of evidence to guide the nurse in planning for and making decisions about care. EBP is an explicit process that facilitates meeting the needs of patients and delivering care that is effective, efficient, equitable, patient-centered, safe, and timely (IOM, 2001).

References

Austin, C. P. (2016). Director's message. National Center for Advancing Translational Sciences. Retrieved from https://ncats.nih.gov/director/message2016

Cochrane, A. L. (1972). *Effectiveness and efficiency: Random reflections on health services*. London: Nuffield Provincial Hospitals Trust. The Cochrane Collaboration.

The Cochrane Collaboration. (2016). Retrieved from http://www.cochrane.org/about-us

Collins, F. S. (2011). Reengineering translational science: The time is right. *Science Translational Medicine, 3*(90), 90cm17.

Dearholt, S., & Dang, D. (2012). *Johns Hopkins Nursing evidence-based practice: Models and guidelines* (2nd ed.). Sigma Theta Tau International, Indianapolis, IN.

Ebsco Publishing. (2016). CINAHL Plus Full Text. Retrieved from http://www.ebscohost.com/academic/cinahl-plus-with-full-text

Estabrooks, C. A. (1998). Will evidence-based nursing practice make practice perfect? *Canadian Journal of Nursing Research, 30*(1), 15–36.

Grady, P. A. (2010). Translational research and nursing science. *Nursing Outlook, 58,* 164–166. doi: 10.1016/j.outlook.2010.01.001

Hanney, S. R., Castle-Clarke, S., Grant, J., Guthrie, S., Henshall, C., Mestre-Ferrandiz, J…Wooding, S. (2015). How long does biomedical research take? Studying the time taken between biomedical and health research and its translation into products, policy, and practice. *Health Research Policy and Systems, 13*(1). doi: 10.1186/1478-4505-13-1

Horsley, J., Crane, J., & Bingle, J. (1978). Research utilization as an organizational process. *Journal of Nursing Administration, 8*(7), 4–6.

Horsley, J. A., Crane, J., Crabtree, M. K., & Wood, D. J. (1983). *Using research to improve nursing practice.* New York: Grune & Stratton.

Institute of Medicine (IOM). (2001). *Crossing the quality chasm: A new health system for the 21st century.* Washington, DC: The National Academies Press.

Institute of Medicine (IOM). (2003). *Health professions education: A bridge to quality.* Washington, DC: The National Academies Press.

Institute of Medicine (IOM). (2010). *The future of nursing: Leading change, advancing health.* Washington, DC: The National Academies Press.

Krueger, J. C. (1978). Utilization of nursing research: The planning process. *Journal of Nursing Administration, 8*(1), 6–9.

Leonenko, M., & Drach-Zahavy, A. (2016). "You are either out on the court, or sitting on the bench": Understanding accountability from the perspectives of nurses and nursing managers. *Journal of Advanced Nursing, 72*(11), 1365–264. doi.org/10.1111/jan.13047

Makary, M. A., & Daniel, M. (2016). Medical error—the third leading cause of death in the U.S. *The BMJ, 35*, 353. doi.org/10.1136

Melnyk, B. M., Gallagher-Ford, L., Long, L. E., & Fineout-Overholt, E. (2014). The establishment of evidence-based practice competencies for practicing registered nurses and advanced practice nurses in real-world clinical settings: Proficiencies to improve healthcare quality, reliability, patient outcomes, and costs. *Worldviews on Evidence-Based Nursing, 11*(1), 5–15. doi:10.1111/wvn.12021

National Library of Medicine. (2016). Retrieved from http://www.nlm.nih.gov/bsd/index_stats_comp.html

Pronovost, P. J. (2010). Learning accountability for patient outcomes. *JAMA, 304*(2), 204–205. doi: 10.1001/jama.2010.979.

Quality and Safety Education for Nurses (QSEN) Institute. (2016) Retrieved from http://www.qsen.org.

U.S. Department of Health and Human Services. (2009). Code of Federal Regulations, Title 45 Public Welfare, Part 46 Protection of Human Subjects. Retrieved from http://www.hhs.gov/ohrp/policy/ohrpregulations.pdf

U.S. Department of Health and Human Services. (2016). Retrieved from http://www.hrsa.gov/quality/toolbox/methodology/qualityimprovement

Critical Thinking and Evidence-Based Practice

The nature of nursing itself compels nurses to play an active role in advancing best practices in patient care. Professional nursing practice involves making judgments; without judgments, nursing is merely technical work (Coles, 2002). Professional judgment is enabled by critical thinking. Critical thinking has many definitions in the literature; however, the complexity of the process requires not only definition but also explanation (Riddell, 2007).

Critical thinking is the complex cognitive process of questioning, seeking information, analyzing, synthesizing, drawing conclusions from available information, and transforming knowledge into action (AACN, 2008). It is a dynamic process, foundational for clinical reasoning and decision-making, and, as such, is an essential component of evidence-based practice (EBP). Every clinical scenario gives the nurse an opportunity to use acquired knowledge and skills to care effectively for the particular individual, family, or group (Dickerson, 2005). Regardless of the nature or source of evidence relating to patient care, critical thinking supplies the necessary skills and cognitive habits needed to support EBP (Profetto-McGrath, 2005).

This chapter describes the knowledge and skills needed to foster critical thinking. The objectives are to describe:

- The similarities among the nursing process, critical thinking, and EBP

- The differences among critical thinking, reasoning, reflection, and judgment

- The way these skills influence evidence appraisal and decisions about applying evidence to practice

- The role of critical thinking in the Practice question, Evidence, and Translation (PET) process

Nursing Process, Critical Thinking, and Evidence-Based Practice

The American Nurses Association (ANA) publication *Nursing: Scope and Standards of Practice* (2004; 2015) references each step of the nursing process, from collection of comprehensive data pertinent to the patient's health or illness through evaluation of the outcomes of planned interventions. It also references integration of the best available evidence, including research findings, to guide practice decisions.

The similarity between EBP and the nursing process is evident: Both are problem-solving strategies. The nursing process structures practice through the following problem-solving stages: assessment, diagnosis, outcome identification, planning, intervention, and evaluation. Although critical thinking is generally considered inherent in the nursing process, this has not been empirically demonstrated (Fesler-Birch, 2005). Nevertheless, the nursing process does require certain skills that are also necessary for critical thinking, such as seeking information and synthesizing it (assessment), drawing conclusions from available information (diagnosis), and transforming knowledge into a plan of action (planning). However, the concept of critical thinking extends beyond this well-defined process.

Paul and Elder (2005) define *critical thinking* as a skill that enables a person to think regularly at a higher level. It transforms thinking in two directions, increasing it systematically and comprehensively. In nursing, Heaslip (2008) views critical thinking for clinical decision-making as the ability to "think in a systematic and logical manner with openness to question and reflect on the reasoning process used to ensure safe nursing practice and quality care. Critical thinking when developed in the practitioner includes adherence to intellectual standards, proficiency in using reasoning, a commitment to develop and maintain intellectual traits of the mind and habits of thought and the competent use of thinking skills and abilities for sound clinical judgments and safe decision-making. To think like a nurse requires that we learn the content of nursing: the ideas, concepts, and theories of nursing and develop our intellectual capacities and skills so that we become disciplined, self-directed, critical thinkers" (p. 1).

Scheffer and Rubenfeld (2000), in their landmark Delphi study of 55 nurse experts in practice, education, administration, and research roles from nine countries, established a consensus definition of critical thinking for nursing:

> Critical thinking in nursing is an essential component of professional accountability and quality nursing care. Critical thinkers in nursing exhibit these habits of mind: confidence, contextual perspective, creativity, flexibility, inquisitiveness, intellectual integrity, intuition, open mindedness, perseverance, and reflection. Critical thinkers in nursing practice the cognitive skills of analyzing, applying standards, predicting and transforming knowledge. (p. 357)

The Johns Hopkins Nursing Evidence-Based Practice (JHNEBP) model's PET process structures the activities of EBP. The nurse asks a focused practice question (P), searches for and appraises relevant evidence (E), and translates the evidence in patient care, evaluating the outcome (T). Each phase requires an analogous set of critical thinking skills including questioning, information seeking, synthesizing, logical reasoning, and transforming knowledge (see Table 2.1).

EBP and what constitutes evidence are continually evolving. Nurses, who are key members of interprofessional teams, participate meaningfully in translating best practices to patient care. Nursing skills that may need strengthening, however, are posing answerable questions, gathering and critically appraising evidence, and determining whether or how to translate relevant findings into practice. These skills are prerequisites to informed decision-making and the application of best practices to the care of patients.

Table 2.1   Alignment of Critical Thinking with the Nursing Process and EBP

Nursing process	Assessment	Diagnosis	Planning, Implementing
Critical thinking	Seek information, and synthesize it	Draw conclusions from available information	Translate knowledge into a plan of action
Evidence-based practice	Pose answerable questions	Search for and appraise relevant evidence	Translate evidence into patient care, and evaluate the outcome

Carper (1978) defined four patterns of knowing in nursing: empirical (the science of nursing), ethical (the code of nursing), personal (knowledge gained from inter-personal relationships between the nurse and the patient), and aesthetic (the art of nursing). Each of these patterns contributes to the body of evidence on which practice is based. Building on Carper's work, McKenna, Cutcliffe, and McKenna (2000) postulated four types of evidence to consider:

- **Empirical:** Based on scientific research
- **Ethical:** Based on the nurse's knowledge of and respect for the patient's values and preferences
- **Personal:** Based on the nurse's experience in caring for the individual patient
- **Aesthetic:** Based on the nurse's intuition, interpretation, understanding, and personal values

The JHNEBP model broadly categorizes evidence as either research or non-research. Scientific (empirical) findings comprise research evidence, whereas non-research evidence includes ethical, personal, and aesthetic evidence. It is the compilation and critical appraisal of all types of evidence, alone and as they relate to each other, that results in the nurse's decision to adopt or reject evidence for use in the care of the individual patient.

Critical Thinking, Reasoning, Reflection, and Judgment

Contemporary nurses are at risk of becoming increasingly task-focused as a result of multiple new technologies, task shifting (Cornell, Riordan, Townsend-Gervis, & Mobley, 2011), and the widespread adoption of electronic health records (EHRs). Time-limited task-focused practice is expected for newly graduated nurses. However, this focus precludes their reflection on the *who, what, where, when,* and *why* of care. Even experienced nurses may fail to ask *why* as they become immersed in managing the diverse and now ever-present technology. EBP not only directs nurses to ask *why* but also guides them in answering questions and making patient-care decisions.

The growing complexity and intensity of patient care demands multiple higher order thinking strategies that include not only critical thinking but also critical reasoning, reflection, and judgment (Benner, Hughes, & Sutphen, 2008, pp. 1–88). Each of these concepts and its applicability to EBP is discussed in Box 2.1.

Whereas critical thinkers strive to develop the ability to make their inferences explicit, along with the assumptions or premises on which those inferences are based, nurses who employ *reasoning* draw conclusions or inferences from observations, facts, or hypotheses. All reasoning has a purpose: It attempts to figure something out, settle a question, or solve a problem. Reasoning is based on assumptions from a specific point of view and on data, information, and evidence expressed through, and shaped by, concepts and ideas. The inferences or interpretations by which one draws conclusions and gives meaning to data have implications and consequences (Paul & Elder, 2005).

| Box 2.1 | Definitions of Critical Thinking, Reasoning, Reflection, and Judgment |

Concept	Definition
Critical thinking	Ability to make inferences explicit, along with the assumptions or premises on which those inferences are based
Reasoning	Drawing conclusions or inferences from observations, facts, or hypotheses
Reflection	Ability to create and clarify the meaning of a particular experience
Judgment	Act of judging or deciding on the basis of reason, evidence, logic, and good sense

Reflection, a key cognitive mechanism in critical thinking, enables nurses to create and clarify the meaning of a particular experience (Forneris & Peden-McAlpine, 2007). Reflection in the context of nursing practice "is viewed as a process of transforming unconscious types of knowledge and practices into conscious, explicit, and logically articulated knowledge and practice that allows for transparent and justifiable clinical decision-making" (Mantzoukas, 2007, p. 7).

Judgment reflects the act of judging or deciding. People have good judgment when they decide on the basis of understanding and good sense. Forming an opinion or a belief, deciding, or acting on a decision is done on the basis of implicit or explicit judgments. To cultivate the ability to think critically, nurses have to develop the habit of judging because of reason, evidence, logic, and good sense (http://www.criticalthinking.org).

Nursing Expertise, Intellectual Competence, and Evidence-Based Practice

In her landmark book *From Novice to Expert: Excellence and Power in Clinical Nursing Practice,* Benner (2001) models the stages of development of clinical expertise in nurses. Progressing from novice to expert, nurses learn to link technical expertise with intuitive expertise. That is, to manage patient-care situations, nurses refine their critical thinking skills to integrate experience with acquired knowledge.

Nursing, in particular, requires specific cognitive skills for excellence in practice; developing these is an essential aspect of their nursing education (Taylor-Seehafer, Abel, Tyler, & Sonstein, 2004). Cognitive skills include:

- **Divergent thinking:** Analyzing a variety of opinions
- **Reasoning:** Differentiating between fact and conjecture
- **Reflection:** Deliberating and identifying multidimensional processes
- **Creativity:** Considering multiple solutions
- **Clarification:** Noting similarities, differences, and assumptions
- **Basic support:** Evaluating credibility of sources of information

Beyond the requisite nursing knowledge and skills, practitioners must have the necessary attitudes, attributes, and habits of mind to use this knowledge appropriately and to complement these skills effectively (Profetto-McGrath, 2005). One approach to defining these dispositions is based on the proposition that certain *intellectual virtues* are valuable to the critical thinker (Foundation for Critical Thinking, 1996). In another approach, *habits of the mind* are identified as exhibited by critical thinkers (Scheffer & Rubenfeld, 2000). These two complementary disposition sets are outlined in Table 2.2. When participating in EBP projects, the team members should be aware of these intellectual virtues and habits to avoid the pitfalls of vague, fragmented, or closed-minded thinking.

Table 2.2   Attributes of Critical Thinkers

Intellectual Virtues of Critical Thinkers	Habits of Mind of Critical Thinkers
■ Intellectual humility: Being aware of the limits of one's knowledge ■ Intellectual courage: Being open and fair when addressing ideas, viewpoints, or beliefs that differ from one's own ■ Intellectual empathy: Being aware of the need to put one's self in another's place to achieve genuine understanding ■ Intellectual integrity: Holding one's self to the same rigorous standards of evidence and proof as one does others ■ Intellectual perseverance: Being cognizant of the need to use rational principles despite obstacles to doing so ■ Faith in reason: Being confident that people can learn to critically think for themselves ■ Fair-mindedness: Understanding that one needs to treat all viewpoints in an unbiased fashion	■ Confidence: Assurance of one's own ability to reason ■ Contextual perspective: Ability to consider the whole in its entirety ■ Creativity: Intellectual inventiveness ■ Flexibility: Capacity to adapt ■ Inquisitiveness: Seeking knowledge and understanding through thoughtful questioning and observation ■ Intellectual integrity: Seeking the truth, even if results are contrary to one's assumptions or beliefs ■ Intuition: Sense of knowing without conscious use of reason ■ Open-mindedness: Receptivity to divergent views ■ Perseverance: Determination to stay on course ■ Reflection: Contemplation for a deeper understanding and self-evaluation

Educating for Critical Thinking Skills

Cultivating critical thinking skills in nursing students and in practicing nurses at all levels is a primary goal for nurse educators and nurse administrators (Shoulders, Follett, & Eason, 2011). Because of the unpredictable nature of patient care, nurses need the ability to analyze and interpret cues, weigh evidence, and respond appropriately and promptly to changing clinical situations, especially those requiring immediate action (Greenwood, Sullivan, Spence, & McDonald, 2000). Furthermore, the ability to think critically is an essential competency for EBP teams when evaluating the cumulative body of evidence for its potential applicability to particular patient-care situations.

Educators can use diverse approaches to structure orientation and training for newly hired nurses, whether experienced or newly graduated. Multiple orientation models can be found in the literature. Educators using the Benner novice-to-expert model may ask: "At what stage would teaching critical thinking and the importance of evidence-based practice be appropriate?" and "When would introducing such skills yield results and benefits for the new nurse/orientee?" The literature suggests that teaching critical thinking and acquiring these skills is best done following the novice stage of development because in the novice stage, nurses are still mastering tasks and procedures. Analysis and reflection, which are critical thinking skills needed for EBP, develop with experience. Other critical thinking skills, however, may increase inquisitiveness, questioning of practice, and inquiry into the best way to apply new knowledge. Encouraging nurses to ask questions allows them to approach their day-to-day care with a clear understanding and a view to improvement.

Critical Thinking and the PET Process

Applying evidence in practice requires a number of steps. The role of critical thinking in each phase of the PET process is described in this section.

Critical Thinking in Posing the Practice Question

In the PET process, the EBP team first defines the scope of the problem by considering the entire situation, including the background and environment relevant to the phenomenon of interest. During this activity, interprofessional team members apply intellectual habits such as confidence, creativity, flexibility, inquisitiveness, intellectual integrity, and open-mindedness. Posing an answerable practice question determines what information to seek and which direction to search. Creating a well-built question often can be more challenging than actually answering the question (Stillwell, Fineout-Overholt, Melnyk, & Williamson, 2010).

The universal intellectual standards cited earlier in this chapter can assist the team in determining the quality of reasoning about a problem, an issue, or a situation (Paul & Elder, 1996) and can help refine the practice question by making it clear, accurate, precise, and relevant. If the question that is posed is unclear or is based on false assumptions, it may not be truly reflective of the issue of concern. If the question is nonspecific, it may not contain sufficient detail to be answerable. If the question is irrelevant to the concern, it could lead to evidence that does not help provide an appropriate answer. The practice question should have enough depth and breadth to reflect the complexities of care but not be so broad that the search for evidence becomes too difficult to manage. Finally, the question needs to make sense and contain no contradictory elements.

Schlosser, Koul, and Costello (2007) proposed identifying and formalizing the process of asking well-built questions to distinguish them from poorly stated questions. The JHNEBP model uses a Question Development Tool (see Appendix B) to serve as a guide for generating useful questions and defining the scope of the problem. Components of this tool as they relate to critical thinking standards are outlined in Table 2.3. The **P**atient, **I**ntervention, **C**omparison, and **O**utcome (PICO) organizing template (Richardson, Wilson, Nishikawa, & Hayward, 1995) can be used to structure question development and is discussed in more detail in Chapter 4.

Table 2.3   Practice Question Development and Critical Thinking Standards

Practice Question Components	Critical Thinking Standards and Questions
What is the practice issue? What is the current practice?	*Clarity:* Is the issue clear? Can we give an example?
How was the practice issue identified?	*Accuracy:* Is it true because we believe it, we want to believe it, we have always believed it, or it is in our best interest to believe it?

Practice Question Components	Critical Thinking Standards and Questions
What are the PICO components? (patient/population/problem, intervention, comparison with other treatments if applicable, outcome)	*Precision:* Can we provide more detail on the issue? What is the issue? What interventions are we questioning? Do we want to compare this with another intervention? *Logic:* What is the desired outcome? Does it really make sense?
State the search question in narrow, manageable terms.	*Precision:* Can we be more specific?
What evidence must be gathered?	*Relevance:* How is this evidence connected to the question? Are we addressing the most significant factors related to the question?
State the search strategy, database, and keywords.	*Breadth:* Do we need to consider other points of view? Are there other ways to look at the question?

Critical Thinking and Appraising Evidence

The evidence phase of the PET process requires proficiency in the following critical thinking skills: seeking information, analyzing, interpreting, and drawing conclusions from available information. The critical analysis, synthesis, and interpretation of evidence are made explicit by the use of rating scales. These standardized levels of evidence facilitate differentiating among varying levels and quality of evidence. The underlying assumption is that recommendations from high levels of evidence and quality would be more likely to represent best practices than lower-level evidence with lesser quality. The rating scale used in the JHNEBP model to determine level and quality of evidence is in Appendix D.

Research evidence has a higher level rating than nonresearch evidence, in particular when the scientific evidence is of high quality. EBP team members apply critical thinking skills when appraising scientific research by focusing on two major components: study design (usually classified as experimental, quasi-experimental, nonexperimental, qualitative, and mixed-methods) and study quality (evaluation of study methods and procedures). When evaluating the summary of overall evidence, teams consider four major components: study design, quality, consistency (similarities in the size and/or direction of estimated effects across studies), and applicability (the extent to which subjects, interventions, and outcome measures are similar to those of interest) (GRADE Working Group, 2004). The various types of research evidence and their associated levels of evidential strength are further explored in Chapter 6.

Because of the complex human and environmental context of patient care, research evidence alone is not sufficient to inform practice. In many instances, scientific evidence either does not exist or is insufficient to shape nursing practice for the individual patient, population, or system. Nonresearch evidence also is needed to inform nursing knowledge and generally includes summaries of research evidence reports, expert opinion, practitioner experience and expertise, patient experience, and human/organizational experience. Clinical appraisal of the level of nonresearch evidence is not as well established as is that for scientific evidence and is therefore more challenging. Because nonresearch evidence is thought to be outside the realm of science and thus less meaningful, appraisal methods have rarely been considered. The various types of nonresearch evidence are discussed in Chapter 7.

The development of any EBP skill set is an evolutionary process. Critical thinking is thought by many to be a lifelong process requiring self-awareness, knowledge, and practice (Brunt, 2005). The JHNEBP model uses a broadly defined quality rating scale to provide structure for the nurse reviewer, yet allows for the application of critical thinking skills specific to the knowledge and experience of the team reviewing the evidence. This scale accommodates qualitative judgments related to both scientific and nonresearch evidence.

Judgments of quality should be continually approached in relative terms. The EBP team assigns a quality grade for each piece of evidence reviewed. The judgment that underlies this determination is in relation to the body of past and present evidence that each member has reviewed. As the group and its individual members gain experience reading and appraising research, their abilities and judgments will likely improve.

Critical Thinking and Translation

The challenge for a nurse participating in an EBP project is translating the contributions of each type of evidence to patient-care decisions. The team must not only grade the level and quality of evidence but also determine the compatibility of recommendations with the patient's values and preferences and the clinician's expertise (Melnyk & Fineout-Overholt, 2006).

Two goals of critical thinking are to assess credibility of information and to work through problems to make the best decisions (Halpern, 1996). This requires flexibility, persistence, and self-awareness. It challenges nurses to consider alternative ways of thinking and acting. Maudsley and Strivens (2000) postulated that a competent practitioner must use critical thinking skills to appraise evidence, tempering realistic notions of scientific evidence with a healthy dose of reflective skepticism. This certainly holds true for nurses as they execute the translation phase of EBP.

Recommendations for Nurse Leaders

Though some key elements of critical thinking are not discussed within the context of the nursing process, some components of critical thinking are clearly vital to the work of nursing. Therefore, nursing accreditation bodies recognize critical thinking as "a significant outcome for graduates at the baccalaureate and master's levels" (Ali, Bantz, & Siktberg, 2005). Furthermore, critical thinking skills such as questioning, analyzing, synthesizing, and drawing conclusions from available information are definite assets to nurses in reaching meaningful evidence-based practice decisions.

Senge (1990) described team learning—the interaction of a team to produce learning and solve problems—as an essential component of learning organizations in which leaders continuously develop capacity for the future. Building capacity for nurses to carry out EBP projects is of strategic importance for nurse leaders; ensuring that nurses have the knowledge and skills required to procure and judge the value of evidence is a top leadership priority.

One way to achieve the successful cultural transition to EBP is to apply the notion of interactive team learning (Sams, Penn, & Facteau, 2004). As members of the EBP team gain experience reviewing and critiquing both research and nonresearch evidence related to a clinical question, their motivation to integrate evidence into practice will increase. Thus, nurses need to have a sound knowledge base regarding the nature of research and nonresearch evidence.

Nurse leaders can best support EBP by providing clinicians with the time, knowledge, and skills necessary to pose answerable questions, to seek and appraise scientific and other quantitative and qualitative evidence within the context of nonresearch evidence, and to make a determination on the advisability of translating evidence into practice. Only through continuous learning and experience can clinicians gain the confidence needed to incorporate the broad range of evidence into the development of protocols and care standards and into the personalized care of the individual patient. Nurse educators also can advance EBP by including related skill development as part of nursing curricula. This can provide a larger pool from which nurse leaders can draw potential employees with a strong educational background in EBP.

Summary

Critical thinking and EBP are inseparable from each other. To take away either one would take away the dynamic, inner core and very life of the other. As nurses sharpen their critical thinking skills, they can more quickly sift the true from the false in the evidence, and the strong points from the weak; and they increase their ability to apply the best evidence available at the time, even where areas of uncertainty may exist. Critically thinking nurses become reflective and maintain an unquenchable spirit of inquiry to bring the best evidence to bear on their practice, thus making their patient care safer and more cost effective and producing better patient outcomes.

Valid clinical questions arise during the course of the nurse's day-to-day patient care activities. These questions form the basis of many EBP projects and benefit from the combined critical thinking of collaborative teams of nurses and their interprofessional colleagues. As Scheffer and Rubenfeld (2006) eloquently stated, "Putting the critical thinking dimensions into the development of evidence-based practice competency demonstrates how critical thinking can be taken out of the toolbox and used in the real world" (p. 195).

References

Ali, N. S., Bantz, D., & Siktberg, L. (2005). Validation of critical thinking skills in online responses. *Journal of Nursing Education, 44*(2), 90–94.

American Association of Colleges of Nursing (AACN). (2008). *The essentials of baccalaureate education for professional nursing practice.* Washington, DC: AACN.

American Nurses Association (ANA). (2004). *Nursing: Scope and standards of practice.* Washington, DC: ANA.

American Nurses Association (ANA). (2015). *Nursing: Scope and standards of practice* (3rd ed.). Silver Spring, MD: American Nurses Association.

Benner, P. E. (2001). *From novice to expert: Excellence and power in clinical nursing practice.* Commemorative Edition. Upper Saddle River, NJ: Prentice Hall.

Benner, P., Hughes, R. G., & Sutphen, M. (2008). Clinical reasoning, decision-making, and action: Thinking critically and clinically. In R. G. Hughes (Ed.). *Patient safety and quality: An evidence-based handbook for nurses* (prepared with support from the Robert Wood Johnson Foundation). AHRQ Publication No. 08-0043. Rockville, MD: Agency for Healthcare Research and Quality, April 2008.

Brunt, B. A. (2005). Critical thinking in nursing: An integrated review. *The Journal of Continuing Education in Nursing, 36*(2), 60–67.

Carper, B. (1978). Fundamental patterns of knowing in nursing. *Advances in Nursing Science, 1*(1), 13–23.

Coles, C. (2002). Developing professional judgment. *Journal of Continuing Education, 22*(1), 3–10.

Cornell, P., Riordan, M., Townsend-Gervis, M., & Mobley, R. (2011). Barriers to critical thinking: Workflow interruptions and task switching among nurses. *Journal of Nursing Administration, 41*(10), 407–414.

Dickerson, P. S. (2005). Nurturing critical thinkers. *The Journal of Continuing Education in Nursing, 36*(2), 68–72.

Fesler-Birch, D. M. (2005). Critical thinking and patient outcomes: A review. *Nursing Outlook, 53*(2), 59–65.

Forneris, S. G., & Peden-McAlpine, C. (2007). Evaluation of a reflective learning intervention to improve critical thinking in novice nurses. *Journal of Advanced Nursing, 57*(4), 410–421.

Foundation for Critical Thinking. (1996). Valuable intellectual virtues. Retrieved from http://criticalthinking.org/resources/articles

GRADE Working Group (2004). Grading quality of evidence and strength of recommendations. *British Medical Journal, 328*(7454), 1490–1498.

Greenwood, J., Sullivan, J., Spence, K., & McDonald, M. (2000). Nursing scripts and the organizational influence on critical thinking: Report of a study of neonatal nurses' clinical reasoning. *Journal of Advanced Nursing, 31,* 1106–1114.

Halpern, D. F. (1996). *Thought and knowledge: An introduction to critical thinking.* Mahwah, NJ: Erlbaun.

Heaslip, P. (2008). Critical thinking and nursing. Retrieved from http://www.criticalthinking.org/pages/critical-thinking-and-nursing/834

Mantzoukas, S. (2007). A review of evidence-based practice, nursing research, and reflection: Leveling the hierarchy. *Journal of Clinical Nursing, 17*(2), 214–223.

Maudsley, G., & Strivens, J. (2000). 'Science,' 'critical thinking', and 'competence' for tomorrow's doctors. A review of terms and concepts. *Medical Education, 34*(1), 53–60.

McKenna, H., Cutcliffe, J., & McKenna, P. (2000). Evidence-based practice: Demolishing some myths. *Nursing Standard, 14*(16), 39–42.

Melnyk, B. M., & Fineout-Overholt, E. (2006). Consumer preferences and values as an integral key to evidence-based practice. *Nursing Administration Quarterly, 30*(2), 123–127.

Paul, R., & Elder, L. (1996). The critical mind is a questioning mind. Retrieved from http://criticalthinking.org/resources/articles

Paul, R., & Elder, L. (2005). *The miniature guide to critical thinking: Concepts and tools.* Dillon Beach, CA: The Foundation for Critical Thinking.

Profetto-McGrath, J. (2005). Critical thinking and evidence-based practice. *Journal of Professional Nursing, 21*(6), 364–371.

Richardson, W. S., Wilson, M. C., Nishikawa, J., & Hayward, R. S. (1995). The well-built clinical question: A key to evidence-based decisions. *ACP Journal Club, 123*(3), A12–A13.

Riddell, T. (2007). Critical assumptions: Thinking critically about critical thinking. *Journal of Nursing Education, 46*(3), 121–126.

Sams, L., Penn, B. K., & Facteau, L. (2004). The challenge of using evidence-based practice. *Journal of Nursing Administration, 34*(9), 407–414.

Scheffer, B. K., & Rubenfeld, M. G. (2000). A consensus statement on critical thinking in nursing. *Journal of Nursing Education*, 39, 352–360.

Schlosser, R. W., Koul, R., & Costello, J. (2007). Asking well-built questions for evidence-based practice in augmentative and alternative communication. *Journal of Communication Disorders*, 40(3), 225–238.

Senge, P. M. (1990). *The fifth discipline: The art and practice of the learning organization.* New York: Doubleday.

Shoulders, B., Follett, C., & Eason, J. (2011). Enhancing critical thinking in clinical practice. *Dimensions of Critical Care Nursing*, 33(4), 207–214.

Stillwell, S. B., Fineout-Overholt, E., Melnyk, B. M., & Williamson, K. M. (2010). Evidence-based practice, step by step: Searching for the evidence. *American Journal of Nursing, 110*(5), 41–47.

Taylor-Seehafer, M. A., Abel, E., Tyler, D. O., & Sonstein, F. C. (2004). Integrating evidence-based practice in nurse practitioner education. *Journal of the American Academy of Nurse Practitioners, 16*(12), 520–525.

# The Johns Hopkins Nursing Evidence-Based Practice Model and Guidelines

The Johns Hopkins Nursing Evidence-Based Practice Model and Process Overview

Evidence-based practice (EBP) is a core competency for all healthcare professionals (IOM, 2003). Using an evidence-based approach to decision-making in healthcare is not only an expectation in healthcare organizations but also a requirement by professional organizations, regulators, health insurers, and purchasers of healthcare insurance. In 2009, the Institute of Medicine (IOM) set a vision that 90% of clinical decisions would be evidence-based by 2020 (IOM, 2009). Because nurses comprise the largest number of healthcare professionals— greater than 3 million—they have the potential to make a major impact on the appraisal and translation of evidence into nursing practice (IOM, 2011; Wilson et al., 2015). To do this requires leaders in both academia and service to align their learning and practice environments to promote healthcare based on evidence, to cultivate a spirit of continuous inquiry, and to translate the highest-quality evidence into practice. Using a model for EBP within an organization fosters end-user adoption of evidence, enables users to speak a common language, standardizes processes, and embeds this practice into the fabric of the organization. The objectives for this chapter are to

- Describe the revised Johns Hopkins Nursing Evidence-Based Practice Model

- Introduce frontline nurses and nurse leaders to the PET (Practice question, Evidence, and Translation) process

Johns Hopkins Nursing Evidence-Based Practice Model—Essential Components: Inquiry, Practice, and Learning

The revised Johns Hopkins Nursing Evidence-Based Practice (JHNEBP) Model (see Figure 3.1) is composed of three interrelated components: inquiry, practice, and learning.

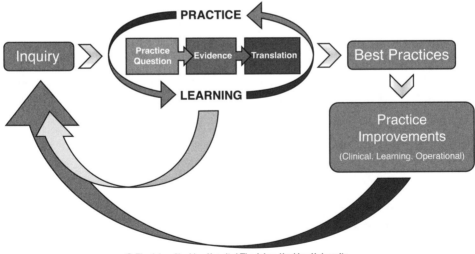

© The Johns Hopkins Hospital/The Johns Hopkins University

Figure 3.1   The Johns Hopkins Nursing Evidence-Based Practice Model (2017).

Inquiry

In the revised JHNEBP Model, inquiry is the initial component that launches the EBP process. The concept of *inquiry,* a foundation for nursing practice, encompasses a focused effort to question, examine, and collect information about a problem, an issue, or a concern. The National League for Nursing (2014) describes a spirit of inquiry as "a persistent sense of curiosity that informs both learning and practice. A nurse motivated by a spirit of inquiry will raise questions, challenge traditional and existing practices, and seek creative approaches to problem-solving … A spirit of inquiry in nursing engenders innovative thinking and extends possibilities for discovering novel solutions in both predictable and unpredictable situations."

Within the practice setting, such inquisitiveness, characterized by an ongoing curiosity about the best evidence to guide clinical decision-making, is what drives EBP (Melnyk, Fineout-Overholt, Stillwell, & Williamson, 2009). Questions about practice commonly arise from nurses' practice settings as they provide everyday care to their patients. These questions may include whether best evidence is being used or whether the care provided is safe, effective, timely, accessible, cost-effective, and high quality. Organizations that foster a culture of inquiry are more likely to have staff that will embrace and actively participate in EBP activities (Melnyk et al., 2009). Nurses have a major impact on building a culture that promotes inquiry by committing to generate and apply new knowledge in practice and to achieve quality outcomes.

Practice

Practice, the basic component of all nursing activity, reflects the translation of what nurses know into what they do. It is the who, what, when, where, why, and how that addresses the range of nursing activities that define the care a patient receives (American Nurses Association [ANA], 2010; ANA, 2015).

Nurses are also bound by, and held to, standards established by professional nursing organizations. For example, the ANA (2015) has identified 6 standards of nursing practice (scope) that are based on the nursing process (see Table 3.1) and 11 standards of professional performance (see Table 3.2). In addition to the

ANA, professional nursing specialty organizations establish standards of care for specific patient populations. Collectively, these standards define nurses' scope of practice, set expectations for evaluating performance, and guide the care provided to patients and families. Because these standards provide broad expectations for practice, all settings where healthcare is delivered must translate these expectations into organization-specific standards such as policies, protocols, and procedures. As part of this process, nurses need to question the basis of their practice and use an evidence-based approach to validate or change current practice based on evidence.

Table 3.1   American Nurses Association Standards of Practice (2015)

Assessment: The collection of comprehensive data pertinent to the healthcare consumer's health or situation. Data collection should be systematic and ongoing. As applicable, evidence-based assessment tools or instruments should be used (for example, evidence-based fall assessment tools, pain rating scales, or wound assessment tools) to identify patterns and variances.

Diagnosis: The analysis of assessment data to determine actual or potential diagnoses, problems, and issues.

Outcomes identification: The identification of expected outcomes for a plan individualized to the healthcare consumer or the situation. The clinician uses clinical expertise and current evidence-based practice to identify health risks, benefits, costs, or the expected trajectory of the condition.

Planning: The development of a plan that prescribes strategies to attain expected measurable outcomes. Includes the development of a plan that is individualized, holistic, and evidence-based and is created in partnership with the healthcare consumer and interprofessional team.

Implementation: Implementation of the identified plan, which includes partnering with the person, family, significant other, and caregivers as appropriate to implement the plan in a safe, effective, efficient, timely, patient-centered, and equitable manner. The clinician utilizes evidence-based interventions and treatments specific to the diagnosis or problem and participates in the translation of evidence into practice. Additionally, the clinician uses evidence-based interventions and strategies to achieve the mutually identified goals and outcomes specific to the problem or needs of the patient.

Evaluation: Progress toward attainment of outcomes. Includes conducting a systematic, ongoing, and criterion-based evaluation of the goals and outcomes in relation to the structures, processes, and timeline prescribed by the plan.

Traditionally, nurses have based their practice on policies, protocols, and procedures that may be unsubstantiated by evidence (Melnyk et al., 2009). However, the use of an evidence-based approach is now an expectation, a standard for the nursing profession, and often a regulatory requirement. For example, healthcare organizations are responding to national healthcare reform by standardizing practices based on evidence in order to reduce inconsistencies in care, and to improve patient safety and quality while reducing healthcare costs (Warren et al., 2016). Evidence-based practice is a prominent aspect of the New Knowledge, Innovations & Improvement component in the Magnet Model (see Figure 3.2). Organizations aspiring to Magnet recognition must show continued growth and expansion of EBP activities, including critical analysis of outcomes and the demonstration of excellence in care delivery (Ingersoll, Witzel, Berry, & Qualls, 2010).

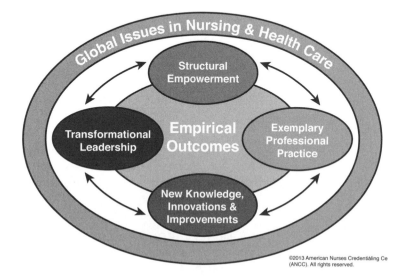

Figure 3.2   American Nurses Credentialing Center Magnet Model components.

Table 3.2   American Nurses Association Standards of Professional Performance (2015)

Ethics: Practicing with compassion and respect for the inherent dignity, worth, and unique attributes of all people. Advocating for the rights, health, and safety of the healthcare of consumers and others. Safeguarding the privacy and confidentiality of healthcare consumers and others and their data and information within ethical, legal, and regulatory parameters.

Culturally congruent practice: Demonstrating respect, equity, and empathy in actions and interactions with all healthcare consumers. Participating in lifelong learning to understand cultural preferences, worldviews, choices, and decision-making processes of diverse consumers.

Communication: Communicating effectively in a variety of formats in all areas of practice.

Collaboration: Collaborating with healthcare consumers, families, and other key stakeholders in the conduct of nursing practice. Partnering with consumers and other key stakeholders to advocate for and effect change, leading to positive outcomes and quality care.

Leadership: Providing leadership in the professional practice setting and the profession. Contributing to the establishment of an environment that supports and maintains respect, trust, and dignity.

Education: Attaining knowledge and competency that reflects current nursing practice and promotes futuristic thinking. Participating in ongoing educational activities. Committing to lifelong learning through self-reflection and inquiry to address learning and personal growth needs.

Evidence-based practice and research: Integrating evidence and research findings into practice by utilizing current evidence-based knowledge, including research findings, to guide practice.

Quality of practice: Contributing to quality nursing practice through quality improvement initiatives, documenting the nursing process in a manner that supports quality and performance improvement, and using creativity and innovation to enhance nursing care.

Professional practice evaluation: Evaluating one's own and others' nursing practice. Providing evidence for practice decisions and actions as part of the formal and informal evaluation processes.

Resource utilization: Utilizing appropriate resources to plan, provide, and sustain evidence-based nursing services that are safe, effective, and fiscally responsible.

Environmental health: Practicing in an environmentally safe and healthy manner. Promoting a safe and healthy workplace and professional practice environment.

The Magnet Model has five key components: (a) transformational leadership; (b) structural empowerment; (c) exemplary professional practice; (d) new knowledge, innovations, and improvements; and (e) empirical outcomes. To provide *transformational leadership*, nursing leaders need to inspire a shared vision, influence, model the way, challenge the process, enable others to act, encourage the heart, and have clinical knowledge and expertise (Wolf, Triolo, & Ponte, 2008). They need to create the vision and the environment that supports EBP activities, such as continuous questioning of nursing practice, translation of existing evidence, and development of new knowledge. Through *structural empowerment*, nursing leaders promote professional staff involvement and autonomy in identifying best practices and using the EBP process to change practice. Magnet organizations demonstrate *exemplary professional practice* such as maintaining strong professional practice models; partnering with patients, families, and interprofessional team members; and focusing on systems that promote patient and staff safety. *New knowledge, innovations, and improvements* challenge Magnet organizations to design new models of care, apply existing and new evidence to practice, and make visible contributions to the science of nursing (American Nurses Credentialing Center [ANCC], 2011). Additionally, organizations are required to have a heightened focus on *empirical outcomes* to evaluate quality. Advanced practice (nurse practitioners, clinical nurse specialists, nurse anesthetists, or nurse midwives) and doctorate of nursing practice (DNP) nurses are vital resources for ensuring a robust EBP process, translating evidence into practice, and evaluating outcomes.

Practice change and improvement will be more readily accepted within the organization and by other disciplines when it is based on evidence that has been evaluated through an interprofessional EBP process. Anecdotal evidence suggests that nursing staff who participate in the EBP process feel a greater sense of empowerment and satisfaction as a result of contributing to changes in nursing practice based on evidence. An organization's ability to create opportunities for nurses as part of an interprofessional team, to develop EBP questions, evaluate evidence, promote critical thinking, make practice changes, and promote professional development is no longer optional.

Learning

According to Braungart, Braungart, and Gramet (2014), "learning is a relatively permanent change in mental processes, emotional functioning, skill, and/or behavior as a result of experience" (p. 64). It is an ongoing informal process of adopting knowledge by applying it in practice that results in a behavior change (Lancaster, 2016). Ultimately, learning is what the learner hears and understands (Holmen, 2014).

A *learning culture* is a culture of inquiry that inspires staff to continuously increase their knowledge and to develop new skills (Linders, 2014; McCormick, 2016). Learning cultures also improve employee engagement, increase employee satisfaction, promote creativity, and encourage problem solving (Nabong, 2015; McCormick, 2016). Both individual learning and a culture of learning are necessary to build practice expertise and maintain staff competency. Education is different from learning in that education imparts knowledge through teaching at a point in time, often in a formal setting. Education makes knowledge available. According to Prabhat (2011), education is largely considered formal and shapes resources from the top down. Formalized education starts with an institution that offers accreditation and then provides resources to meet that expressed goal. In contrast, learning begins with individuals and communities. The desire to learn, a natural desire, is often considered informal learning and is based on the interests of individuals or groups, who access resources in pursuit of that interest.

Ongoing learning is necessary to remain current with new knowledge, technologies, and skills, and to establish clinical competencies. Learning also serves to inform practice, which leads to changes in care standards that drive improvements in patient outcomes. Because the field of healthcare is becoming increasingly more complex and technical, no single individual can know everything about how best to provide safe and effective care, and no single degree can provide the knowledge needed to span an entire career. It is, therefore, an essential expectation that nurses participate in lifelong learning and continued competency development (IOM, 2011).

"Education is what people do to you. Learning is what you do for yourself."

–Joi Ito

Lifelong learning is not only individual learning but also interprofessional, collaborative, and team-oriented learning. For example, joint learning experiences between nursing and medical students can facilitate a better understanding of roles and responsibilities, make communication more effective, aid in conflict resolution, and foster shared decision-making. Joint learning can also improve collaboration and the ability to work more effectively on interprofessional EBP teams. The use of interprofessional education and learning fosters collaboration in implementing clinical standards, improving services, and preparing teams to solve problems using an EBP approach that exceeds the capacity of any lone professional (IOM, 2011).

The JHNEBP Model—Description

Inquiry is the starting point for using the JHNEBP Model (refer to Figure 3.1 on page 36). An individual or a team, sparked by genuine curiosity, seeks to identify whether current practice reflects the best evidence for a specific problem or a particular patient population. The PET process provides a systematic approach for solving a practice question, finding the best evidence, and translating best evidence into practice. As the individual or team moves through the PET process, they are continually learning by gaining new knowledge, improving skills in collaboration, and gaining insights. At any point in the learning-and-practice cycle, insights can trigger a new EBP process. Practice changes can also trigger additional learning as specific practice settings and patient populations are considered. These improvements are often clinical, learning, or operational in nature. As a result, the PET process informs both practice and learning, which prompts behavior changes to improve practice through the use of best evidence. This ongoing cycle of inquiry, practice, and learning and identifying best evidence and implementing practice improvements makes the JHNEBP model a dynamic and interactive process for practice changes that are likely to impact system, nurse, and patient outcomes.

Factors Impacting the JHNEBP Model

The JHNEBP Model (2017) is an open system with interrelated components. Because it is an open system, inquiry, learning, and practice are influenced by not only evidence but also factors external and internal to the organization. External factors can include accreditation bodies, legislation, quality measures, regulations, and standards. Accreditation bodies (e.g., The Joint Commission, Commission on Accreditation of Rehabilitation Facilities) require an organization to achieve and maintain high standards of practice and quality. Legislative and regulatory bodies (local, state, and federal) enact laws and regulations designed to protect the public and promote access to safe, quality healthcare services. Failure to adhere to these laws and regulations has adverse effects on an organization, most often financial. Examples of regulatory agencies are the Centers for Medicare & Medicaid Services, Food and Drug Administration, and state boards of nursing. State boards of nursing regulate nursing practice and enforce the Nurse Practice Act, which serves to protect the public. Quality measures (outcome and performance data) and professional standards serve as yardsticks for evaluating current practice and identifying areas for improvement or change. The American Nurses Credentialing Center, through its Magnet Recognition Program, developed criteria to assess the quality of nursing and nursing excellence in organizations. Additionally, many external stakeholders such as healthcare networks, special interest groups/organizations, vendors, patients and their families, the community, and third-party payors exert influence on healthcare organizations.

Internal factors can include organizational culture, values, and beliefs; practice environment (e.g., leadership, resource allocation, patient services, organizational mission and priorities, availability of technology, library support, time to conduct EBP activities); equipment and supplies; staffing; and organizational standards. Enacting EBP within an organization requires

- A culture that believes EBP will lead to optimal patient outcomes
- Strong leadership support at all levels with the necessary resources (human, technological, and financial) to sustain the process
- Clear expectations that incorporate EBP into standards and job descriptions
- Development of EBP mentors such as unit-based EBP champions, and advanced practice and DNP nurses to serve as teachers and role models and to assist with EBP team leadership
- A culture that supports interprofessional collaboration

Partnerships and interprofessional collaboration are crucial for the implementation of EBP initiatives that are in alignment with a healthcare organization's mission, goals, and strategic priorities (Moch, Quinn-Lee, Gallegos, & Sortedahl, 2015). Knowledge and evaluation of the patient population and the internal and external factors that impact the healthcare institution are essential for successful implementation and sustainability of EBP within an organization.

JHNEBP PET Process: Practice Question, Evidence, and Translation

The 19-step JHNEBP process (see Appendix A) occurs in three phases and can be simply described as PET (see Figure 3.3). The process begins with the identification of a practice problem, issue, or concern. This step is critically important because how the problem is posed drives the remaining steps in the process. Based on the problem statement, a *practice question* is developed and refined, and a search for *evidence* is conducted. The evidence is then appraised and synthesized. Based on this synthesis, the team makes a determination of whether the evidence supports a change in practice. If the data supports a change, evidence *translation* begins and the practice change is planned, implemented, and evaluated. The final step in translation is the dissemination of results to patients and their families, staff, hospital stakeholders, and, if appropriate, the local and national community.

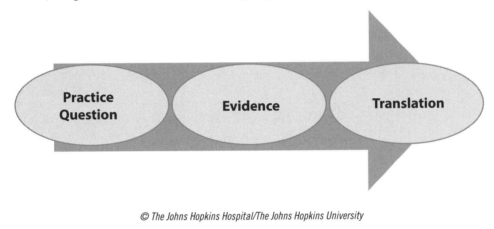

© *The Johns Hopkins Hospital/The Johns Hopkins University*

Figure 3.3   JHNEBP PET process.

Practice Question

The first phase of the process (Steps 1–6) includes forming a team and developing an answerable EBP question. An interprofessional team examines a practice concern and develops and refines an EBP question. Refer to the Project Management Guide (see Appendix A) frequently throughout the process to direct the team's work and gauge progress. The tool identifies the following steps.

Step 1: Recruit interprofessional team

The first step in the EBP process is to form an interprofessional team to examine a specific practice concern. It is important to recruit members for which the question holds relevance. When members are interested and invested in addressing a specific practice concern, they are generally more effective as a team. Front-line clinicians are key members because they likely have firsthand knowledge of the problem, its context, and its impact. Other relevant stakeholders may include team members such as clinical specialists (nursing or pharmacy), members of committees or ancillary departments, physicians, dieticians, pharmacists, patients, and families. These stakeholders provide discipline-specific expertise or insights to create the most comprehensive view of the problem and, thus, the most relevant practice question. Keeping the group size to 6–8 members makes it easier to schedule meetings and helps to maximize participation.

Step 2: Define the problem

It is essential that the team take the necessary time to carefully determine the problem accurately. The team needs to identify the gap between the current practice and the desired practice—in other words, between what the team actually sees and experiences and what they want to see and experience. The team should state the question in different ways and get feedback from nonmembers to see whether there is agreement on the problem statement. Teams should spend time on gathering information, both narrative and numerical, to identify why the current practice is a problem. Team members should also observe the practice and listen to how actual users describe the issues related to the problem. It is helpful for team members to visualize what the current practice looks like in contrast to future practice requirements. The time devoted to probing issues and challenging assumptions about the problem, looking at it from multiple angles and obtaining feedback from as many sources as possible, is always time well spent. Incorrectly identifying the problem results in wasted effort searching and appraising evidence that, in the end, does not provide the insight that allows the team to achieve the desired outcomes.

Step 3: Develop and refine the EBP question

The next step is to develop and refine the clinical, learning, or operational EBP question (see Appendix B). Keeping the EBP question narrowly focused makes the search for evidence specific and manageable. For example, the question "What is the best way to stop the transmission of methicillin-resistant staphylococcus aureus (MRSA)?" is extremely broad and could encompass many interventions and all practice settings. This type of question, known as a *background question,* is often used when the team knows little about the area of concern or is interested in identifying best practices. In contrast, a more focused question is, "What works best in the critical-care setting to prevent the spread of MRSA—hand washing with soap and water or the use of alcohol-based hand sanitizers?" This type of question, known as a *foreground question*, is generally used by more experienced teams with specialized knowledge to compare interventions or make decisions. In general, foreground questions are narrow and allow the search for evidence to be more precise and focused.

The PET process uses the PICO mnemonic (Sackett, Straus, Richardson, Rosenberg, & Haynes, 2000) to describe the four elements of a focused question: (a) patient, population, or problem, (b) intervention, (c) comparison with other treatments, and (d) measurable outcomes (see Table 3.3).

Table 3.3   Application of PICO Elements

*P*atient, population, or problem

Team members determine the specific patient, population, or problem related to the patient/population/issue under examination. Clinical examples include age, ethnicity, disease, and setting. Nonclinical examples include timeliness, effectiveness, efficiency, and patient centeredness.

*I*ntervention

Team members identify the specific intervention process or approach to be examined. Examples include treatments, protocols, education, self-care, and best practices.

*C*omparison with other interventions, if applicable

Team members identify what they are comparing the intervention to—for example, current practice or intervention.

*O*utcomes

Team members identify expected outcomes based on the implementation of the practice change. The outcomes (measures) include rate-based and nonrate-based metrics that will determine the effectiveness if a change in practice is implemented.

The Question Development Tool (see Appendix B) guides the team in defining the practice problem, examining current practice, identifying how and why the problem was selected, limiting the scope of the problem, and narrowing the EBP question using the PICO format. The tool also helps the team develop a search strategy by identifying the sources of evidence to be searched and possible search terms. It is important to recognize that the EBP team can go back and further refine the EBP question as more information becomes known as a result of the evidence search and review. Refer to Chapter 4 for more details regarding the development and refining of an EBP practice question.

Step 4: Identify stakeholders

It is important for the EBP team to identify early the appropriate individuals and stakeholders who should be involved in, and kept informed during, the EBP project. A *stakeholder* is a person, group, or department in an organization that has an interest in, or a concern about, the topic or project under consideration (Agency for Healthcare Research and Quality, 2011). Stakeholders may include a variety of clinical and nonclinical staff, departmental and organizational leaders, patients and families, regulators, insurers, or policy makers. Keeping key stakeholders informed is instrumental to successful change. The team should consider whether the EBP question is specific to a unit, service, or department or involves multiple departments. If it is the latter, representatives from all areas involved need to be recruited for the EBP team. Key leadership in the affected departments should be kept up-to-date on the team's progress. If the problem affects multiple disciplines (e.g., nursing, medicine, pharmacy, respiratory therapy), each discipline should also be included. The Stakeholder Analysis Tool (see Appendix C) can be used to guide stakeholder identification.

Step 5: Determine responsibility for project leadership

Identifying a leader for the EBP project facilitates the process, accountabilities, and responsibilities and keeps the project moving forward. The leader should be knowledgeable about EBP and have experience and a proven track record in leading interprofessional teams. It is also helpful if this individual knows the organizational structure and strategies for implementing change within the organization.

Step 6: Schedule team meetings

Setting up the first EBP team meeting includes such activities as

- Reserving a room with adequate space conducive to group discussion
- Asking team members to bring their calendars so that subsequent meetings can be scheduled
- Ensuring that a team member is assigned to record discussion points and group decisions
- Establishing a timeline for the process
- Keeping track of important items (e.g., copies of the EBP tools, literature searches, materials, and resources)
- Providing a place to keep project files

Evidence

The second phase (Steps 7–11) of the PET process addresses the search for, appraisal of, and synthesis of the best available evidence. Based on these results, the team makes recommendations regarding practice changes.

Step 7: Conduct internal and external search for evidence

Team members determine what type of evidence to search for (see Chapter 5), who is to conduct the search, and who will bring items to the committee for review. Enlisting the help of a health information specialist (librarian) is critical. Such assistance saves time and ensures a comprehensive and relevant search. In addition to library resources, other sources of evidence include

- Clinical practice guidelines
- Community standards

- Opinions of internal and external experts
- Organizational financial data
- Position statements from professional organizations
- Patient and staff surveys and satisfaction data
- Quality improvement data
- Regulatory, safety, or risk management data

Step 8: Appraise the level and quality of each piece of evidence

In this step, research and nonresearch evidence is appraised for level and quality. The Research Evidence Appraisal Tool (see Appendix E) and the Nonresearch Evidence Appraisal Tool (see Appendix F) assist the team in this activity. Each tool includes a set of questions to determine the type, level, and quality of evidence. The PET process uses a 5-level scale to determine the level of the evidence, with Level I evidence as the highest and Level V as the lowest (see Appendix D). Based on the questions provided on the tools, the quality of each piece of evidence is rated as high, good, or low-major flaws. The team reviews each piece of evidence and determines both the level and the quality. Evidence with a quality rating of low-major flaws is discarded and is not used in the process. The Individual Evidence Summary Tool (see Appendix G) tracks the team's appraisal of each piece of evidence (including the author, date, evidence type, sample, sample size, setting, and study findings), which helps to answer the EBP question and identify the limitations, level, and quality of evidence. Chapters 6 and 7 provide a detailed discussion of evidence appraisal.

Step 9: Summarize the individual evidence

The team numerically sums the evidence documents that answer the practice question for each level of evidence and records the totals on the Synthesis Process and Recommendations Tool (see Appendix H). The relevant findings that answer the EBP question for each level are then written in summary form next to the appropriate level.

Step 10: Synthesize overall strength and quality of evidence

Through synthesis, the team makes a determination of the overall strength and quality of the collected body of evidence, taking into consideration the (a) level, (b) quality, (c) quantity, (d) consistency of findings across all pieces of evidence, and (e) applicability to the population and setting. The team can use the quality criteria for individual evidence appraisal as a guide for determining overall quality. Making decisions about the overall strength is both an objective and a subjective process. The EBP team should devote the necessary time to thoughtfully evaluate the body of evidence and come to agreement on the overall strength. Refer to Chapters 6 and 7 and Appendix H for more information on evidence synthesis.

Step 11: Develop recommendations for change based on evidence synthesis

Based on the overall appraisal and synthesis of the evidence, the team considers possible pathways to translate evidence into practice. A team has four common pathways to consider when developing a recommendation (Poe & White, 2010):

- Evidence may be compelling, with consistent results that support a practice change.

- Evidence may be good, with consistent results that support a practice change.

- Evidence may be good, but with conflicting results that may or may not support a practice change.

- Evidence may be nonexistent or insufficient to support a practice change.

Based on the selected translation pathway, the team then determines whether to make the recommended change or investigate further (see Table 3.4). The team lists its recommendations on the Synthesis Process and Recommendations Tool (see Appendix H). Carefully consider the risks and benefits of making the change. We strongly recommended piloting changes in several representative areas/settings to determine possible unanticipated effects or barriers.

Table 3.4   Translation Pathways for EBP Projects

	Evidence			
	Compelling, consistent	**Good, consistent**	**Good but conflicting**	**Insufficient/ absent**
Make recommended change?	Yes	Consider pilot of change	No	No
Need for further investigation?	No	Yes, particularly for broad application	Yes, consider periodic review for new evidence or development of research study	Yes, consider periodic review for new evidence or development of research study
Risk-benefit analysis	Benefit clearly outweighs risk	Benefit may outweigh risk	Benefit may or may not outweigh risk	Insufficient information to make determination

Reprinted from Poe and White (2010)

Translation

In the third phase (Steps 12–19) of the process, the EBP team determines whether the changes to practice are feasible and appropriate and are a good fit given the target setting. If they are, the team creates an action plan, implements and evaluates the change, and communicates the results to appropriate individuals both internal and external to the organization.

Step 12: Determine fit, feasibility, and appropriateness of recommendation(s) for translation pathway

The team communicates and obtains feedback from appropriate organizational leaders, bedside clinicians, and all other stakeholders affected by the practice recommendations to determine whether the change is feasible and appropriate and is a good fit for the specific practice setting. Team members examine the risks and benefits of implementing the recommendations. They must also consider the resources available and the organization's readiness for change (Poe & White, 2010). Even with strong, high-quality evidence, EBP teams may find it difficult to implement practice changes in some cases. For example, an EBP team examined the best strategy for ensuring appropriate enteral tube placement after initial tube insertion. The evidence indicated that x-ray was the only 100% accurate method for identifying tube location. The EBP team recommended that a post-insertion x-ray be added to the enteral tube protocol. Despite their presenting the evidence to clinical leadership and other organizational stakeholders, the team's recommendation was not accepted within the organization. Concerns were raised about the additional costs and adverse effects that may be incurred by patients (appropriateness). Other concerns related to delays in workflow and the availability of staff to perform the additional x-rays (feasibility). Risk management data showed a lack of documented incidents related to inappropriate enteral tube placement. As a result, after weighing the risks and benefits, the organization decided that making this change was not a good fit at that time. The fit-and-feasibility section of the Synthesis Process and Recommendations Tool (see Appendix H) provides a list of questions to consider when determining both fit and feasibility.

Step 13: Create action plan

If the recommendations are a good fit for the organization, the team develops a plan to implement the practice change(s). The plan may include

- Development of (or change to) a standard (policy, protocol, guideline, or procedure), a critical pathway, or a system or process related to the EBP question

- Development of a detailed timeline assigning team members to the tasks needed to implement the change (including the evaluation process and reporting of results)

- Solicitation of feedback from organizational leaders, bedside clinicians, and other stakeholders.

Essentially, the team must consider the *who, what, when, where, how,* and *why* when developing an action plan for the proposed change. The Action Planning Tool (see Appendix I) provides a guide for the EBP team to develop the action plan.

Step 14: Secure support and resources to implement action plan

The team needs to give careful consideration to the human, material, or financial resources needed to implement the action plan. Obtaining support and working closely with departmental and organizational leaders can help to ensure the successful implementation of the EBP action plan.

Step 15: Implement action plan

When the team implements the action plan, they need to ensure that all affected staff and stakeholders receive verbal and written communication as well as education about the practice change, implementation plan, and evaluation process. EBP team members should be available to answer any questions and troubleshoot problems that may arise during implementation.

Step 16: Evaluate outcomes

Using the outcomes identified on the Question Development Tool (see Appendix B), the team evaluates the degree to which the outcomes were met. Although the team desires positive outcomes, unexpected outcomes often provide opportunities for learning, and the team should examine why these occurred. This examination may indicate the need to alter the practice change or the implementation process, followed by reevaluation.

It is also important to note that information from which inferences can be made about the EBP project's outcomes can fall under one of three categories: structure, process, or outcomes (Donabedian, 1988). *Structure* refers to the setting in which care is provided and may include, for example, (a) material resources such as facilities, equipment, and money; (b) human resources, such as the number and qualification of personnel; and (c) organizational characteristics such as culture, peer review, shared governance, policies, and protocols. *Process* refers to what is actually being done when providing care (e.g., patient care activities, interaction between patients and providers of care), and *outcomes* refers to the effects of care on the health status of the patient or the effectiveness of the intervention. EBP teams need to recognize the linkage between all three categories when assessing the results of an EBP project. According to Donabedian (1988), if good structures are in place, it increases the likelihood of a good process, which in turn increases the likelihood of good outcomes. As a result, understanding the relationship between all three categories is important to the final analysis of the end results of the EBP project, particularly if the results are less than expected. Upon completion of the evaluation process, if the decision is made to continue the practice change, the organization's quality improvement process should be undertaken when ongoing measurement, evaluation, and reporting are indicated.

Step 17: Report outcomes to stakeholders

In this step, the team reports the results to appropriate organizational leaders, frontline clinicians, and all other stakeholders. Sharing the results, both favorable and unfavorable, helps disseminate new knowledge and generates additional practice or research questions. Valuable feedback obtained from stakeholders can overcome barriers to implementation or help develop strategies to improve unfavorable results. The Dissemination Tool (see Appendix J) guides the EBP team in identifying the audience(s), key message points, and methods to communicate the team's findings, recommendations, and practice changes.

Step 18: Identify next steps

EBP team members review the process and findings and consider whether any lessons have emerged that should be shared or whether additional steps need to be taken. These lessons or steps may include a new question that has emerged from the process, the need to do more research on the topic, additional training that may be required, suggestions for new tools, the writing of an article on the process or outcome, or the preparation of an oral or poster presentation at a professional conference. The team may identify other problems that have no evidence base and, therefore, require the development of a research protocol. For example, when the recommendation to perform a chest x-ray to validate initial enteral tube placement was not accepted (see the example discussed in Step 12), the EBP team decided to design a research study to look at the use of colorimetric carbon dioxide detectors to determine tube location.

Step 19: Disseminate findings

This final step of the process is one that is often overlooked and requires strong organizational support. The results of the EBP project need to be, at minimum, communicated to the organization. Depending on the scope of the EBP question and the outcome, consideration should be given to communicating findings external to the organization in appropriate professional journals or through presentations at professional conferences. Refer to the Dissemination Tool (see Appendix J).

Summary

This chapter introduces the revised JHNEBP Model (2017) and the steps of the PET process. Nursing staff with varied experience and educational preparation have successfully used this process with mentorship and organizational support. They have found it rewarding both in understanding the basis for their current nursing interventions and incorporating changes into their practice based on evidence (Dearholt & Dang, 2012).

References

Agency for Healthcare Research and Quality. (2011). Engaging stakeholders to identify and prioritize future research needs. Retrieved from http://www.effectivehealthcare.ahrq.gov/index.cfm/search-for-guides-reviews-and-reports/?pageaction=displayproduct&productid=698

American Nurses Association (ANA). (2010). *Nursing: Scope and standards of practice*. Washington, DC: American Nurses Association.

American Nurses Association (ANA). (2015). *Nursing: Scope and standards of practice* (3rd ed.). Silver Spring, MD: American Nurses Association.

American Nurses Credentialing Center (ANCC). (2011). Announcing the model for ANCC's magnet recognition program. Retrieved from http://www.nursecredentialing.org/Magnet/ProgramOverview/New-Magnet-Model.aspx

Braungart, M., Braungart, R. G., & Gramet, P. R. (2014). Applying learning theories to healthcare practice. In S. B. Bastable (Ed.), *Nurse as Educator, Principles of Teaching and Learning for Nursing Practice* (pp. 64–110), Burlington, MA: Jones & Bartlett Learning.

Dearholt, S. L., & Dang, D. (2012). *Johns Hopkins nursing evidence-based practice: Model and guidelines* (2nd ed.). Indianapolis, IN: Sigma Theta Tau International.

Donabedian, A. (1988). The quality of care: How can it be assessed? *JAMA, 260*(12), 1743–1748.

Holmen, M. (2014, August 6). Education vs learning—what exactly is the difference [Web log post]. *EdTechReview.* Retrieved from http://edtechreview.in/trends-insights/insights/1417-education-vs-learning-what-exactly-is-the-difference?utm_content=buffer4e5b8&utm_medium=social&utm_source=twitter.com&utm_campaign=buffer#.U-NdPce3yG4.twitter

Ingersoll, G. L., Witzel, P. A., Berry, C., & Qualls, B. (2010). Meeting Magnet research and evidence-based expectations through hospital-based research centers. *Nursing Economics, 28*(4), 226–235.

Institute of Medicine (IOM). (2003). *Health professions education: A bridge to quality.* Washington, DC: National Academics Press.

Institute of Medicine (IOM). (2009). Roundtable on evidence-based medicine. Washington, DC: National Academies Press. Retrieved from https://www.ncbi.nlm.nih.gov/books/NBK52847

Institute of Medicine (IOM). (2011). *The future of nursing: Leading change, advancing health.* Washington, DC: The National Academics Press.

Lancaster, J. (2016). Changing health behavior using health education with individuals, families, and groups. In M. Stanhope & J. Lancaster (Eds.), *Public Health Nursing* (355–376). St. Louis, MO: Elsevier Mosby.

Linders, B. (2014). Nurturing a culture for continuous learning. *InfoQ.* Retrieved from https://www.infoq.com/news/2014/07/nurture-culture-learning

McCormick, H. (2016). Seven steps to creating a lasting learning culture. University of North Carolina. Retrieved from http://www.kenan-flagler.unc.edu/~/media/Files/documents/executive-development/unc-white-paper-7-steps-to-creating-a-lasting-learning-culture

Melnyk, B. M., Fineout-Overholt, E., Stillwell, S. B., & Williamson, K. M. (2009). Igniting a spirit of inquiry: An essential foundation for evidence-based practice. *American Journal of Nursing, 109*(11), 49–52.

Moch, S. D., Quinn-Lee, L., Gallegos, C., & Sortedahl, C. K. (2015). Navigating evidence-based practice projects: The faculty role. *Nursing Education Perspectives, 36*(2), 128–130.

Nabong, T. (2015). Creating a learning culture for the improvement of your organization. *Training Industry.* Retrieved from https://www.trainingindustry.com/workforce-development/articles/creating-a-learning-culture-for-the-improvement-of-your-organization.aspx

National League for Nursing. (2014). Practical/vocational nursing program outcome: Spirit of inquiry. Retrieved from http://www.nln.org/docs/default-source/default-document-library/spirit-of-inquiry-final.pdf?sfvrsn=0

Poe, S. S., & White, K. M. (2010). *Johns Hopkins Nursing Evidence-Based Practice: Implementation and Translation*. Indianapolis, IN: Sigma Theta Tau International.

Prabhat, S. (2011, July 28). Difference between education and learning. *Difference Between*. Retrieved from http://www.differencebetween.net/miscellaneous/difference-between-education-and-learning

Sackett, D. L., Straus, S. E., Richardson, W. S., Rosenberg, W., & Haynes, R. B. (2000). *Evidence-based medicine: How to practice and teach EBM*. Edinburgh: Churchill.

Warren, J. I., McLaughlin, M., Bardsley, J., Eich, J., Esche, C. A., Kropkowski, L., & Risch, S. (2016). The strengths and challenges of implementing EBP in healthcare systems. *Worldviews on Evidence-Based Nursing, 13*(1), 15–24.

Wilson, M., Sleutel, M., Newcomb, P., Behan, D., Walsh, J., Wells, J. N., Baldwin, K. M. (2015). Empowering nurses with evidence-based practice environments: Surveying Magnet, Pathway to Excellence, and non-Magnet facilities in one healthcare system. *Worldviews on Evidence-Based Nursing, 12*(1), 12–21.

Wolf, G., Triolo, P., & Ponte, P. R. (2008). Magnet recognition program: the next generation. *Journal of Nursing Administration*, 38(4), 200–204.

III

Practice Question, Evidence, Translation (PET)

The Practice Question

Practice questions frequently arise from day-to-day problems encountered by clinicians, administrators, and nurse educators. Answers to these questions in the form of evidence are available in print or by way of electronic media or evidence summaries such as systematic reviews, integrative reviews, literature reviews, and guidelines. The objectives of this chapter are:

- Identify the steps in forming an EBP team
- Define practice problems appropriate for an EBP approach
- Use the PICO framework to create an answerable EBP question

The practice question phase of the PET process (Practice question, Evidence, Translation) includes six operational steps, shown in Box 4.1. The first step is to assemble an interprofessional team to examine a specific practice concern or problem. Team members work together to define and develop a comprehensive understanding of the problem, followed by refinement of the evidence-based practice (EBP) question, identification of stakeholders, selection of a project leader, assignment of team responsibilities, and development of the meeting schedule. The Johns Hopkins Nursing Evidence-Based Practice (JHNEBP) Question Development Tool (see Appendix B) facilitates this phase.

Box 4.1   Steps in Practice-Question Phase—the *P* in PET Process

Step 1: Recruit interprofessional team

Step 2: Define the problem

Step 3: Develop and refine the EBP question

Step 4: Identify the stakeholders

Step 5: Determine the responsibility for project leadership

Step 6: Schedule the team meetings

The Interprofessional EBP Team

Having interprofessional representation on the EBP team is critical to the team's success. The range of disciplines of team members depends on the focus and scope of the problem. For example, if the problem is postoperative hypothermia management, representatives from anesthesia and surgery should be included. Anticipating whose practice may be affected determines which individuals or groups should be involved either as team members or as stakeholders. The EBP team members should have expertise relevant to the problem under consideration. Usually, the team includes nurses, physicians, and other professional staff who contribute significantly or are knowledgeable of the problem. For example, if the question relates to best practices in the management of nausea for the patient undergoing chemotherapy, the team may consist of nurses, pharmacists, and oncologists.

The number of members should be small enough to promote efficiency and be large enough to provide content expertise—typically, six to eight people. Consider involving a patient as a stakeholder or team member for patient-centered problems. Team members' responsibilities are to attend meetings, review and present evidence, participate in evidence synthesis, generate practice recommendations, and contribute to and support team decisions. Teams that have never conducted an EBP project can benefit by recruiting an experienced mentor to help them complete the process the first time.

After the team is assembled and ready to begin the PET process, members select a team leader. This leader should be someone who can facilitate meetings, manage projects, articulate the team's recommendations, and influence implementation. The leader engages team members to establish a regular meeting schedule so that members can adjust their schedules ahead of time. Selecting a time and venue away from the demands of the clinical area and within a timeline realistic enough to complete the project is essential. Team members who work multiple shifts, on various days, and in different roles often require as much as two months' notice. Occasionally, teams with regularly scheduled meetings established for quality improvement, policy and procedure review, or other professional responsibilities use a portion of this standard meeting time for the EBP project.

Some teams schedule a preliminary meeting to refine the practice problem and question and then one or two 8-hour days to review evidence and make recommendations. Others have approached scheduling challenges by setting aside 4-hour blocks of time monthly or five 2-hour meetings every other week. Scheduling meetings weekly or every two weeks keeps the team moving forward. Delays between group meetings diminish the team's momentum.

Defining Practice Problems

Interprofessional team members begin their task by defining the practice problem. Defining the problem precisely and succinctly is important because all subsequent actions and decisions build on the clarity and accuracy of the problem statement. The process often begins by seeking answers to practice concerns such as:

- Is there evidence that this intervention works?
- How does this practice help the patient?

- Why are we doing this practice, and should we be doing it this way?
- Is there a way to improve this practice so that it is more efficient or more cost-effective?
- How can we improve the quality, safety, and cost of our practice?

Practice problems can emerge from multiple sources. Titler et al., in two classic publications (1994, 2001), identified problem-focused or knowledge-focused triggers as sources of problems. *Problem-focused triggers* are those identified by staff during routine monitoring of quality, risk, financial, or benchmarking data or adverse events. *Knowledge-focused triggers* are identified by reading published reports or learning new information at conferences or professional meetings (see Table 4.1).

Table 4.1   Sources of Evidence-Based Practice Problems

Trigger	Sources of Evidence-Based Practice Problems
Problem-focused	Financial concerns
	Evidence for current practice questioned
	Quality concern (efficiency, effectiveness, timeliness, equity, patient-centeredness)
	Safety or risk management concerns
	Unsatisfactory patient, staff, or organizational outcomes
	Variations in practice compared with external organizations
	Variations in practice within the setting

Trigger	Sources of Evidence-Based Practice Problems
Knowledge-focused	New sources of evidence
	Changes in standards or guidelines
	New philosophies of care
	New information provided by organizational standards committees

Problems may also be recurring or priority issues within an organization or a practice that has questionable benefit. Clinical questions can seek to help nurses understand dissimilar outcomes between two patient populations. Why do some patients in the intensive care unit (ICU), for example, develop ventilator-associated pneumonia whereas other ICU patients do not? There may be a difference in practice among nurses, nursing units, or peers outside of the organization. The potential for problems to generate practice questions is limitless, and EBP projects have the potential to result in improvements in health, organization of systems, or education. Problems that are important are those that can cause harm, result in an unsatisfactory experience, or diverge or vary from established standards of care or that are associated with high resource use (e.g., staffing or costs). With the advent of value-based purchasing, healthcare teams and organizations are now financially rewarded or penalized for performance on quality and safety outcomes, preventable adverse conditions, and costs. Thus, it is crucial that EBP teams, before beginning the EBP project, consider and select problems that align with identified priorities within their organization. When time and effort are dedicated to only those questions that are important, potential benefits accrue to patients, nurses, and organizations, such as:

- Increased visibility of nursing leadership and contributions
- New levels of support from clinicians and organizational leaders
- Tangible quality and safety benefits to patients and families
- Values-based organizational outcomes

A robust problem statement provides a comprehensive understanding of the population of interest (e.g., patients, nurses, families, and their characteristics) and how they are affected (e.g., of 24 surgical patients that were in the supine position for more than 4 hours, five developed pressure ulcers on their heels). Precise descriptions clarify the scope and magnitude of the problem related to the outcome of interest. Discussion of the problem enables the interprofessional team to reflect, gather information, observe current practice, listen to clinicians, visualize how the process can be different or improved, and probe the description—together fostering a shared understanding. Proceeding without a clear problem statement results in:

- EBP questions that do not address the problem

- Searches that are too broad and lead the team to review more evidence than is needed to answer the question

- Missing evidence that is important to answer the question, because specific and sensitive search terms were not used

- Team frustration with the effectiveness of the EBP process

A number of strategies can be used to help define problems. For example, phrasing the problem statement in terms of the knowledge gap rather than the solution or asking clarifying questions (e.g., where, why, when, how) allows the team to probe deeper into the nature or root cause of the problem. Table 4.2 provides specific strategies for defining the problem and shows an example of each one. Time spent defining the problem clearly and concisely facilitates the construction of a good EBP question.

Table 4.2   Strategies for Defining the EBP Problem

Strategy	Examples	Rationale
Phrase the problem statement in terms of the knowledge gap, not the solution.	Knowledge gap *Staff lack knowledge of the best strategies to manage patient pain immediate post-discharge total knee replacement* Solution *Patients need a better pain management strategy for the immediate post-discharge period.*	Allows the team to see other, potentially more effective, solutions
State the problem rather than symptoms of the problem.	Problem *40% of patients discharged post total knee replacement complain that they were not able to manage their pain.* Symptom *Patients with total knee replacement were not satisfied after discharge.*	Allows the team to determine the true problem, and its size and scope, without being sidetracked by outward signs that a problem exists
Describe in precise terms the perceived gap between what one sees and what one wants to see.	Current State *Patient satisfaction with pain management post discharge is 36%.* Future State *This is compared to a national benchmark of 85%.*	Allows the team to assess the current state and envision a future state in which broken components are fixed, risks are prevented, new evidence is accepted, and things that were missing elements are provided

continues

Table 4.2   Strategies for Defining the EBP Problem   (continued)

Strategy	Examples	Rationale
Examine the problem critically, and make sure that the final statement defines the specific problem.	Specific problem *Do patients understand their pain management regimen?* Assumed problem *Are patients following the prescribed pain management regimen?*	Gives the team time to gather information, observe, listen, and probe to ensure a true understanding of the problem
Ask clarifying questions.	Clarifying questions *When are these patients experiencing pain?* *What are the precipitating factors?* *How often are they taking their pain medications?*	Helps the team get to the specific problem by using question words such as *when, what, how*
Refrain from blaming the problem on external forces or focusing attention on the wrong aspect of the problem.	Attributing blame *The patients are noncompliant with the prescribed pain-medication therapy.* *The nurses did not educate the patient properly about the importance of taking pain medications as prescribed.*	Keeps the team focused on processes and systems as the team moves to define the EBP question
State the problem in a different way.	Restating problem *40% of patients with post total knee replacement had low patient satisfaction scores related to pain management after discharge.*	Helps gain clarity by using different verbs

Strategy	Examples	Rationale
Challenge assumptions.	Is the team's assumption correct? *The patient fills the pain-medication prescription and is taking pain medication in the way that it was prescribed.*	Helps the team avoid conjecture and question everyday processes and practices that are taken for granted
Expand and contract the problem.	Expanded problem *Is dissatisfaction with post-discharge pain management part of a general dissatisfaction with the hospital stay as a whole?* Contracted problem *Are there multiple reasons for dissatisfaction with post-discharge pain management, such as inability to pay for pain medications or fear of becoming dependent on pain medications?*	Helps the team understand whether the problem is part of a larger problem or is made up of many smaller problems
Assume multiple solutions.	Multiple solutions *What ARE best practices for managing post-discharge pain in patients following total knee replacement?* Single solution *What IS the best practice for managing post-discharge pain in patients following total knee replacement?*	Helps the team identify more than one possible solution to determine the best fit for the population of interest

Developing Answerable EBP Questions

Having agreed on the nature and scope of the practice problem, the EBP team develops an answerable question that addresses a clinical, administrative, or knowledge problem (see Appendix B).

EBP projects require time, availability of evidence, EBP skills, expert mentors, and leadership support. Consequently, the EBP model and process may not be practical for all questions. Choose questions that have a high return on quality and safety outcomes as well as those that align with organizational priorities. Before embarking on an EBP project and committing the necessary time and resources, consider the following questions:

- Would the practice changes resulting from this project improve clinical or staff outcomes, unit structures or processes, or patient or nurse satisfaction?

- Would they reduce the cost of care?

- Can potential practice changes be implemented given the current culture, practices, and organizational structure within the particular practice setting?

Choosing a Background or Foreground Question

There are two types of EBP questions: background and foreground (Sackett, Rosenberg, Gray, Haynes, & Richardson, 1996; Sackett, Straus, Richardson, Rosenberg, & Haynes, 2000). A *background question* is a best practice question that is broad and produces a wide range of evidence for review. Background questions are used to identify and understand what is known when the team has little knowledge, experience, or expertise in the area of interest (e.g., concept, treatment, intervention). For example, a background question intended to better understand pain management for people with a history of substance abuse is as follows: *What are the best nursing interventions to manage pain for patients with a history of substance abuse?* This question would produce evidence related to pharmacology, alternative therapies, behavioral contracting, and biases in prescribing and administering pain medication. Evidence identified for background questions often provides a large number of studies with diverse populations, settings, and interventions.

Foreground questions yield specific knowledge that informs decisions or actions and generally compare two or more specific interventions. In some instances, the information gained from background questions can be used to develop foreground questions. The following is an example of a foreground question: *Is behavioral contracting or mutual goal setting more effective in improving the chronic-pain experience for adult patients enrolled in outpatient rehabilitation with a history of substance abuse?* Foreground questions produce a refined, limited body of evidence specific to the EBP question. In this example, a narrow patient population is added (adults enrolled in outpatient rehabilitation with a history of substance abuse), the nature of pain specified (chronic), and intervention comparison identified (mutual goal setting versus behavioral contracting).

One important point to note is that when an EBP team is asking a background question, the evidence review can become complex. As a result, it may be helpful to organize the EBP project by breaking down the components of the problem into an appropriate number of foreground questions. To do this, the team could create questions that relate to each of the components identified. For example, if the problem is high fall rates in older inpatients, the background question could be, *What are the best practices in fall prevention for older patients?* An appropriate foreground question could be, *Which practice is more effective in reducing fall-related injury in older adults: bed alarms or hourly rounding?*

Figure 4.1 depicts the relationship between background and foreground questions. Teams with little experience with a topic or condition will have more background questions (A), whereas teams with more experience with the condition will generally have more foreground questions (C). Often, EBP teams will benefit from a thorough understanding of the background of an issue before diving into the more specific foreground issues (DiCenso, Guyatt, & Ciliska, 2005). As their understanding and experience with the topic or issue deepens, they move into more focused foreground questions (B).

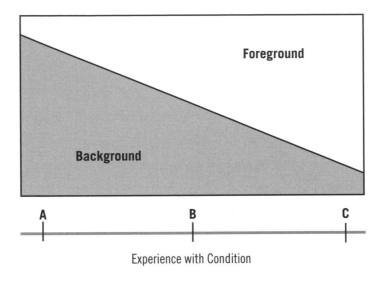

Figure 4.1   Background and foreground questions.

Sackett, Straus, Richardson, Rosenberg, & Haynes, 2000)

Developing an Answerable EBP Question

The thoughtful development of a well-structured EBP question is important because the question drives the strategies used to search for evidence. Making the
EBP question as specific as possible helps to identify and narrow search terms,
which, in turn, reduces time spent searching for relevant evidence and increases
the likelihood of finding it. Creating a specific question focuses the EBP project
and provides a sensitive evidence review that accurately addresses the problem
and question. It is also useful for defining the target population, such as age, gender, ethnicity, diagnosis, and procedure, so that translation of the recommendations is planned appropriately. (Chapter 5 describes using keywords for evidence
searches.)

Richardson, Wilson, Nishikawa, & Hayward (1995) published a helpful format
for constructing an answerable EBP question that is referred to as PICO—
Patient, Population or Problem, Intervention, Comparison, and Outcome. PICO
frames the problem clearly and facilitates the evidence retrieval by identifying
key search terms.

*P*atient, population, or problem

Describe the patient, population, or problem succinctly. Include the type of patient or population and the setting. Consider patient attributes such as age, gender, symptoms, and diagnosis (patient's problem) or issues such as effectiveness, timeliness, efficiency, or safety.

*I*ntervention

The intervention can be a treatment; a clinical, learning, or operational intervention; or a structure or process of care (see definitions and examples in Table 4.3).

*C*omparison with other intervention(s)

Determine if a comparison intervention exists. Will this intervention be compared to another? Not all questions have comparisons, particularly if you are asking a background question. A statement of current practice may be used as a comparison.

*O*utcomes

Define measures that will be used to determine the effect of the intervention on target population (e.g., readmission, quality of life, hand hygiene, compassion fatigue. Once the measure(s) is defined, the next step is to describe how it will be calculated (the metric). A *metric* is the degree to which a particular subject possesses the quality that is being measured. Measures can be rate-based or nonrate-based. Rate-based metrics are calculated using a numerator and denominator. For example, if the outcome of interest is patient falls, the metric will describe how falls will be measured. In this example, the metric would be the total number of falls (numerator) per 1,000 patient days (denominator). Nonrate-based measures are counts or frequency of occurrence or a process measure such as symptom experience. Measuring outcomes indicates the level of success in achieving the desired outcome(s). A measurement plan (see Appendix B) guides teams through this process.

Table 4.3   Definitions and Examples of Structures, Processes, and Outcomes of Care

Concept	Definition	Examples
Structure	Attributes of the setting	Adequacy of facility, equipment, and staff; qualifications of staff; availability of resources; policies
Process	Any patient care activity or intervention	Hand washing, aseptic technique; triage algorithms in the emergency department; medication administration
Outcome	Effects of care on health status and populations	Quality of life, patient satisfaction, surgical site infection

Source: Donabedian, 1988

Table 4.4 provides an example using PICO to create a foreground question. The question is, *For adult surgical inpatients between the ages of 20 and 50 with a peripheral intravenous catheter, does the use of saline to flush the peripheral IV maintain IV patency and decrease phlebitis over 48 hours when compared to heparin flushes?*

Table 4.4   PICO Example of a Foreground Question

P—Patient, population, or problem	Adult surgical inpatients (patients) between the ages of 20 and 50 years old with a peripheral intravenous catheter (population)
I—Intervention	Use of saline flushes
C—Comparison	Use of heparin flushes for peripheral IV maintenance
O—Outcomes	Improvements in IV patency over 48 hours (process) and decrease in the incidence of phlebitis by 10% (outcome)

Scope of Project, Stakeholders, and Designating Responsibility

After the problem is stated and the question created, the team reassesses whether other stakeholders should be involved and determines the EBP project lead, team members, and responsibilities.

The team will start by identifying whether the problem is clinical, learning, or operational and describing the current practice. Describing the current practice helps in three ways:

1. Clarifies specific processes that may be the source of the problem

2. Establishes baseline data

3. Indicates how much of a change will be required when recommendations are made prior to translation

The selection of appropriate stakeholders is based on who is affected by the problem or concern, where is it experienced, and when it occurs. Answering these questions influences who needs to be added to the team, informed, or involved.

The EBP team leader will need to designate responsibility for the subsequent steps in the EBP process. Action items may include inviting new members to the team, reporting to internal committees, or providing information to organizational leaders about the EBP project.

Summary

This chapter introduces the multiple origins of practice problems appropriate for an EBP approach. It is essential to begin this first stage of the EBP project systematically with an interprofessional team to define the problem and to generate an EBP question using the PICO format. Team members will determine whether other stakeholders should be included or informed and designate team members' responsibility. The ultimate goal of the *P* in the PET process is a well-framed practice question to guide the next phase of the EBP process, (Evidence) successfully and efficiently.

References

DiCenso, A., Guyatt, G., & Ciliska, D. (2005). *Evidence-based nursing: A guide to clinical nursing.* St. Louis: Elsevier Mosby.

Donabedian, A. (1988). The quality of care: How can it be assessed? *JAMA, 260,* 1743–1748.

Richardson, W. S., Wilson, M. C., Nishikawa, J., & Hayward, R. S. (1995). The well-built clinical question: A key to evidence-based decisions. *American College of Physicians, 123*(3), A12–A13.

Sackett, D. L., Rosenberg, W. M., Gray, J. A., Haynes, R. B., & Richardson, W. S. (1996). Evidence based medicine: What it is and what it isn't. *British Medical Journal, 312*(7023), 71–72.

Sackett, D. L., Straus, S. E., Richardson, W. S., Rosenberg, W., & Haynes, R. B. (2000). *Evidence-based medicine: How to practice and teach EBM.* Edinburgh: Churchill.

Titler, M. G., Kleiber, C., Steelman, V., Goode, C., Rakel, B., Barry-Walker, J.,...Buckwalter, K. (1994). Infusing research into practice to promote quality care. *Nursing Research, 43*(5), 307–313.

Titler, M. G., Kleiber, C., Steelman, V. J., Rakel, B. A., Budreau, G., Everett, L. Q., ...Goode, C. J. (2001). The Iowa model of evidence-based practice to promote quality care. *Critical Care Nursing Clinics of North America, 13*(4), 497–509.

Searching for Evidence

Developing information literacy skills requires knowledge of the nursing literature and an aptitude for locating and retrieving it. "Given the consistent need for current information in health care, frequently updated databases that hold the latest studies reported in journals are the best choices for finding relevant evidence to answer compelling clinical questions" (Hartzell, Fineout-Overholt, Hofstetter, & Ponder, 2015, p. 43). Studies have shown that positive changes in a nurse's information literacy skills and increased confidence in using those skills have a direct impact on appreciation and application of research, are vital for effective lifelong learning, and are a prerequisite to evidence-based practice, or EBP (McCulley & Jones, 2014).

Evidence can be collected from a variety of sources, including the World Wide Web and proprietary databases. The information explosion has made it difficult for healthcare clinicians, researchers, educators, administrators, and policy makers to process all the relevant literature available to them every day. Evidence-based clinical resources, however, have made searching for medical information much easier and faster than in years past. This chapter:

- Describes key information formats
- Identifies steps to find evidence to answer the EBP questions
- Suggests information and evidence resources
- Provides tips for search strategies
- Suggests methods of evaluating search results

Key Information Formats

Nursing is awash with research data and resources in support of evidence-based nursing, which itself is continually evolving (Johnson, 2015). Evidence-based literature comes from many sources, and nurses need to keep them all in mind. The literature search is a vital component of the EBP process. If nurses search only a single resource, database, or journal, they will likely miss important evidence. Through the search, nurses expand their experience in locating evidence important to the care they deliver.

Translation literature refers to evidence-based research findings that, after much research and analysis, have been translated into guidelines used in the clinical setting. It includes practice guidelines, protocols, standards, critical pathways, clinical innovations, evidence-based care centers, peer-reviewed journals, and bibliographic databases. Some sources of translation literature are the National Guideline Clearinghouse, the Best Practice information sheets of the Joanna Briggs Institute, the Cumulative Index to Nursing and Allied Health Literature (CINAHL), and PubMed. (Information on accessing such resources is provided later in this chapter.)

Evidence summaries include systematic reviews, integrative reviews, meta-analysis, meta-synthesis, and evidence synthesis. These are summaries of the literature that identify, select, and critically appraise relevant research and use appropriate statistical or interpretive analysis to summarize the results of the studies. Evidence-based summaries can be found in library catalogs, online book collections, and online resources such as PubMed, CINAHL, the Cochrane Library, and the Joanna Briggs Institute. For hospital administrators and case managers, Health Business FullText is a source for quality improvement and financial information.

Primary evidence is data generally collected from direct patient or subject contact and includes hospital data, clinical trials, peer-reviewed research journals, conference reports and abstracts, and monographs, as well as summaries from data sets such as the Centers for Medicare & Medicaid Services (CMS) Minimum Data Set. Databases where this information can be found include PubMed, CINAHL, Excerpta Medica Database (EMBASE), library catalogs, and institutional repositories. For hospital administrators, the Healthcare Cost and Utilization Project (HCUP) is a source for health statistics and information on hospital inpatient and emergency department use.

The Answerable Question

After a practice problem has been identified and converted into an answerable EBP question (see Chapter 4), the search for evidence begins with the following steps:

1. Identify the searchable keywords contained in the EBP question and list them on the Question Development Tool (see Appendix B). Include also any synonymous or related terms.

2. Identify the types of information needed to best answer the question and list the sources where such information can be found. What database(s) will provide the best information to answer the question?

3. Develop the search strategy.

4. Evaluate search results for relevance to the EBP question.

5. Revise the search strategy as needed.

6. Record the strategy specifics (terms used, limits placed, years searched) on the Question Development Tool and save the results.

EBP Search Examples

The first step in finding evidence is selecting searchable keywords from the answerable EBP question. The Question Development Tool facilitates this process by directing the team to identify the practice problem and, using the PICO components, to develop the search question.

For example, consider the following background question: "What risk factors are associated with serious injury from falls in the adult acute care setting?" Some search terms to use may be *falls*, *risk factors*, *adults*, and *acute care settings*. Table 5.1 illustrates how the PICO format focuses these terms. However, additional terms such as *hospitals*, *injury*, *ambulatory care facilities*, and terms synonymous or linked to fall prevention could also be used.

Table 5.1   PICO Example: Risk Factors Associated with Injury from Falls

P (Patient, population, problem):	Adults in acute-care settings
I (Intervention):	Identification of fall-injury risk factors
C (Comparison):	(Not applicable)
O (Outcomes):	Decrease in serious injury from falls

Teams need to consider the full context surrounding the problem when thinking of search terms. As an example, *intervention* is a term used frequently in nursing; it encompasses the full range of activities a nurse undertakes in the care of patients. Searching the literature for *nursing interventions*, however, is far too general and needs to be focused on specific interventions. In the preceding example, "Risk Factors Associated with Injury from Falls," possible interventions may include *medication*, *equipment*, and *floor coverings*. Table 5.2 shows the development of an answerable background question for a specific EBP problem and the corresponding search strategy.

Table 5.2   Search Strategy for Distractions and Interruptions During Medication Administration

Problem
A hospital's quality improvement committee saw an increase in medication errors, and nurses indicated that distractions and interruptions were the largest contributing factor. Unit staff did not know what the best strategies were for controlling distractions and interruptions in their work environment during the medication administration process.

PICO	
P (Patient, population, problem):	Nurses on inpatient-care units
I (Intervention):	Identification and control of distractions and interruptions in environment during medication administration
C (Comparison):	(Not applicable)
O (Outcomes):	Decrease in distractions and interruptions

Answerable Question
"What are the best practices to help nurses on inpatient units recognize and control interruptions and distractions during the medication administration process?"

Initial Search Terms	Related Search Terms
Hospital personnel	Nurses, physicians
Distractions	Health personnel
Medication errors	Attention, interruptions
Medication administration	

Selecting Information and Evidence Resources

After search terms have been selected, EBP teams can identify quality databases containing information on the topic. This section briefly reviews some of the unique features of core EBP databases in nursing and medicine.

CINAHL

The CINAHL covers nursing, biomedicine, alternative or complementary medicine, and 17 allied health disciplines. CINAHL indexes more than 3,100 journals, contains more than 3.4 million records dating back to 1981, and has complete coverage of English-language nursing journals and publications from the National League for Nursing and the American Nurses Association (ANA). In addition, CINAHL contains healthcare books, nursing dissertations, selected conference proceedings, standards of practice, and book chapters. Full-text material within CINAHL includes more than 70 journals in addition to legal cases, clinical innovations, critical paths, drug records, research instruments, and clinical trials.

CINAHL also contains a controlled vocabulary, *CINAHL Subject Headings,* which allows for more precise and accurate retrieval. Terms are searched using "MH for Exact Subject Heading" or "MM for Exact Major Subject Heading." CINAHL also allows you to search using detailed limits to narrow results by publication type, age, gender, and language. The PICO on distractions could be searched using the CINAHL headings (MH "Distraction") AND (MH "Medication Errors") in combination with the keywords *distraction* and *medication errors.* The search strategy would look like this: ((MH "Distraction") OR distraction) AND ((MH "Medication Errors") OR "medication errors").

MEDLINE and PubMed

MEDLINE and PubMed are often used interchangeably; however, teams need to keep in mind that they are *not* the same. PubMed searches MEDLINE but also searches articles that are not yet indexed in MEDLINE and articles that are included in PubMed Central.

MEDLINE, available for free through the National Library of Medicine's interface, PubMed, contains over 26 million references to journal articles in the life sciences with a concentration on biomedical research. One of MEDLINE's most notable features is an extensive, controlled vocabulary: *Medical Subject Headings (MeSH)*. Each record in MEDLINE is reviewed by an indexer who is a specialist in a biomedical field. The indexer assigns an appropriate MeSH heading to every record, which allows for precise searching by eliminating irrelevant articles where a keyword may be casually mentioned. A common saying in the library world is: "Garbage in, garbage out." MeSH can eliminate "garbage," or irrelevant articles.

To search in PubMed using the PICO example for distractions during medication administration, one would use the MeSH for "Medication Errors" [MeSH]. MeSH has no term for "distractions," but *distraction* as a keyword can be used. The related MeSH term of "Attention" [MeSH] could also be considered. The search strategy would look like this: ("Medication Errors"[MeSH] OR "medication errors"[All Fields]) AND ("Attention"[MeSH] OR distraction [All Fields]).

PubMed also contains *Clinical Queries*, which has prebuilt evidence-based filters. Clinical Queries uses these filters to find relevant information on topics relating to one of five clinical study categories: therapy, diagnosis, etiology, prognosis, and clinical prediction guides. Clinical Queries also includes a search filter for systematic reviews. This filter combines search terms with a filter that limits results to systematic reviews, meta-analyses, reviews of clinical trials, evidence-based medicine, consensus development conferences, and guidelines.

The Cochrane Library

The Cochrane Library is a collection of databases that most notably includes the Cochrane Database of Systematic Reviews. Internationally recognized as the gold standard in evidence-based health care, Cochrane Reviews investigate the effects of interventions for prevention, treatment, and rehabilitation. They also assess the accuracy of a diagnostic test for a given condition in a specific patient group and setting. Over 6,900 Cochrane Reviews are currently available and as many as 2,450 protocols. Abstracts of reviews are available free of charge from the Cochrane website; full reviews require a subscription. A medical librarian can identify the organization's access to this library.

Joanna Briggs Institute (JBI)

The *Joanna Briggs Institute (JBI)* is an international, not-for-profit, membership-based research and development organization. Part of the Faculty of Health Sciences at the University of Adelaide, South Australia, they collaborate internationally with over 70 entities. The Institute and its collaborating entities promote and support the synthesis, transfer, and utilization of evidence by identifying feasible, appropriate, meaningful, and effective practices to improve healthcare outcomes globally. JBI includes *Best Practice information sheets* that are produced specifically for health professionals and are based on evidence reported in systematic reviews. The JBI resources and tools are available only by subscription through Ovid, and a medical librarian can identify the organization's access to this resource.

Selecting Resources Outside of the Nursing Literature

At times it may become necessary to expand searches beyond the core nursing literature. Databases typically related to nursing research and practice are briefly presented in this section.

PsycINFO

PsycINFO is a database supported by the American Psychological Association that focuses on research in psychology and the behavioral and social sciences. PsycINFO contains more than 4 million records, including journal articles, book chapters, book reviews, editorials, clinical case reports, empirical studies, and literature reviews. The controlled vocabulary for PsycINFO is available through the Thesaurus feature. Thesaurus terms can be searched as major headings and can be exploded to search for terms that are related and more specific. Searches in PsycINFO can be limited by record type, methodology, language, and age to allow for a more targeted search.

Health and Psychosocial Instruments (HaPI)

The HaPI database contains approximately 190,000 records for scholarly journals, books, and technical reports. HaPI is produced by the Behavioral Measurement Database Services and provides behavioral measurement instruments for use in the nursing, public health, psychology, social work, communication, sociology, and organizational behavior fields.

Physiotherapy Evidence Database (PEDro)

The Physiotherapy Evidence Database (PEDro) is a free resource that contains over 33,000 citations for randomized trials, systematic reviews, and clinical practice guidelines for physiotherapy. The Center for Evidence-Based Physiotherapy at the George Institute for Global Health produces this database and attempts to provide links to full text, when possible, for each citation in the database.

Creating Search Strategies and Utilizing Free Resources

In the following section we will cover the necessary components used to create a solid search strategy. Databases are unique, so the components you select when creating a search strategy will vary; not every search strategy will utilize every component. The end of this section includes a list of free, reliable resources with descriptions explaining the content available in each resource. Remember to check with your local medical library to see what additional resources may be available to you.

Key Components to Creating Search Strategies

After appropriate resources are identified to answer the question, the EBP team can begin to create a search strategy. Keep in mind that this strategy needs to be adjusted for each database. Begin by breaking the question into concepts, selecting keywords and phrases that describe the concepts, and identifying appropriate, controlled vocabulary. Use *Boolean operators* (*AND, OR*, and *NOT*) to combine or exclude concepts. Remember to include spelling variations and limits where necessary. Note that the search strategies for PubMed and CINAHL in the previous sections were created by combining the AND and OR Boolean operators.

Use OR to combine keywords and controlled vocabulary related to the same concept: ("Attention" [MeSH] OR distraction). Use AND to combine two separate concepts: ("Attention" [MeSH] OR distraction) AND ("Medication Errors" [MeSH] OR "medication errors").

Review the following steps to build a thorough search strategy:

1. Use controlled vocabularies when possible. Controlled vocabularies are specific terms used to identify concepts within an index or database. They are important tools because they ensure consistency and reduce ambiguity where the same concept may have different names. Additionally, they often improve the accuracy of keyword searching by reducing irrelevant items in the retrieval list. Some well-known vocabularies are MeSH in MEDLINE (PubMed) and CINAHL Subject Headings in CINAHL.

2. Use the Boolean operators. Boolean operators are AND, OR, and NOT. Use OR to combine keywords and phrases with controlled vocabulary. Use AND to combine each of the concepts within your search. Use NOT to exclude keywords and phrases; use this operator with discretion to avoid excluding terms that are relevant to the topic. (See Figure 5.1.)

Boolean Operator Example	Venn Diagram
"Attention" [MeSH] **AND** "Medication Errors" [MeSH] Articles that have both terms, *attention* and *medication* errors	
"Attention" [MeSH] **OR** distraction Articles that have the terms *attention* only or *distraction* only or both terms	
distraction **NOT** "Osteogenesis, Distraction" [Mesh] Articles with the term *distraction*, excluding *osteogensis* or articles with *distractions* and *osteogensis*	

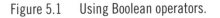

Figure 5.1   Using Boolean operators.

3. Use alternative spellings to create an exhaustive search. Remember that even within the English language, you have spelling variations in American and British literature. In British literature, *Ss* often replace *Zs*, and *OUs* often replace *Os*. Two examples of this are *organisation* versus *organization* and *behaviour* versus *behavior*.

4. Use limits where appropriate. Most databases have extensive limits pages. PubMed and CINAHL allow you to limit by age, gender, species, date of publication, and language. The limit for publication types assists in selecting the highest levels of evidence: meta-analysis, practice guidelines, randomized controlled clinical trials, and controlled clinical trials.

5. Revise your search. As you move through steps 1–4, you are likely to find new terms, alternate spellings of keywords, and related concepts. You need to revise your search to incorporate these changes. Your search is only complete when you can answer your question. If you were given a previous search to update, you will need to make revisions, because terms may have changed over time and new related areas of research may have developed.

Free Resources

Most databases require a paid subscription, but some are available for free online. Table 5.3 lists quality resources available for free on the Internet. Check the local medical or public library to see what is accessible. Medical librarians, knowledgeable about available resources and how each functions, can assist in the search for evidence and can provide invaluable personalized instruction. Never be afraid to ask for help! The only foolish question is the one unasked.

Table 5.3   Free Online Resources

Resource	Focus	Website
National Guideline Clearinghouse (NGC)	Practice Guidelines	http://www.guideline.gov
NIH RePORTER: Research Portfolio Online Reporting Tool	Federally Funded Research Projects	http://report.nih.gov
PubMed	Biomedical Research	http://www.ncbi.nlm.nih.gov/sites/entrez?db=PubMed
PubMed Central Homepage	Full-Text Biomedical Resources	http://report.nih.gov
PubMed Health	Clinician and Consumer Information	http://www.ncbi.nlm.nih.gov/pubmedhealth
Registry of Nursing Research: Virginia Henderson International Nursing Library	Research and Conference Abstracts	http://www.nursinglibrary.org/portal/main.aspx
The Cochrane Collaboration	Systematic Reviews	http://report.nih.gov
Turning Research into Practice (TRIP) Database: For Evidence-Based Medicine (EBM)	Clinical Practice	http://www.tripdatabase.com/index.html
US Preventive Services Task Force (USPSTF)	Clinician and Consumer Information	http://www.uspreventiveservicestaskforce.org
Google Scholar	Multidisciplinary Resources	http://scholar.google.com

The *NGC* is a federal government resource that contains practice guidelines. NGC is available free of charge from the Agency for Healthcare Research and Quality (AHRQ); its mission is to provide a resource for objective, detailed information on clinical practice guidelines. The database includes summaries about the guidelines, links to full texts where available, and a guidelines comparison chart.

The National Institutes of Health (NIH) *RePORTER* is a federal government database that lists biomedical research projects funded by the NIH as well as the Centers for Disease Control and Prevention (CDC), AHRQ, Health Resources and Services Administration (HRSA), Substance Abuse and Mental Health Services Administration (SAMHSA), and U.S. Department of Veterans Affairs (VA). RePORTER allows extensive field searching, hit lists that can be sorted and downloaded in Microsoft Excel, NIH funding for each project (expenditures), and publications and patents that have acknowledged support from each project (results).

PubMed Health is a free database from the National Center for Biotechnology Information (NCBI) at the U.S. National Library of Medicine (NLM). PubMed Health provides information on the prevention and treatment of diseases and conditions. Resources are focused on reviews of clinical effectiveness research for clinicians and easy-to-read summaries for consumers.

The *Virginia Henderson International Nursing Library*, a service offered through the Honor Society of Nursing, Sigma Theta Tau International, offers nurses online access to reliable information that can be easily utilized and shared. The library's complimentary *Registry of Nursing Research* database allows searches of both study and conference abstracts. Primary investigator contact information is also available for requests of full-text versions of studies.

The *TRIP* is a clinical search tool designed to allow health professionals to rapidly identify the highest-quality evidence for clinical practice. It searches hundreds of evidence-based medicine and nursing websites that contain synopses, clinical answers, textbook information, clinical calculators, systematic reviews, and guidelines.

USPSTF was created in 1984 as an independent volunteer panel of national experts in prevention and EBM. It works to improve health by making evidence-based recommendations on clinical preventive services such as screenings, counseling services, and preventive medications, drawing from preventive medicine and primary care including family medicine, pediatrics, behavioral health, obstetrics and gynecology, and nursing.

Google Scholar is a free resource that allows a broad search across many disciplines and sources for scholarly literature. It contains articles, theses, books and abstracts, and court opinions. Sources for content come from academic publishers, professional societies, online repositories, universities, and other websites. Nonmedical terms can be used, and due to its multidisciplinary nature, content can be accessed related to non-nursing subject matter. Google Scholar ranks documents by weighting the full text, publisher, and author(s), as well as how recently and frequently it has been cited in other scholarly literature.

Though Google Scholar can be simple to use because of its familiarity and the wide use of Google as a search engine, the EBP team must be cautious. Not all journals are indexed, and search algorithms change daily, making it impossible to replicate a search. As with any database, the EBP team must realize that searching using only Google Scholar will result in insufficient evidence (Bramer, Giustini, & Kramer, 2016). With these caveats in mind, the EBP team can enjoy some additional benefits when using Google Scholar.

If the EBP team is not associated with a hospital or academic library, they may not have access to online databases. Google Scholar remains free and open to the public. A helpful feature is the user's ability to set up routine alerts for relevant search terms and have them emailed. For example, if the EBP team is searching the literature using search terms *fall risk* and *acute care*, a recommendation rule can be set up so that any time a new scientific document is added, an email can be sent directly to the EBP team, alerting them to this information. Finally, Google Scholar has the ability to export citations to certain bibliography managers (for example, RefWorks, RefMan, EndNote, and BibTeX) to help keep track of references.

The team can also gain valuable information by searching the table of contents of subject-related, peer-reviewed journals and by evaluating the reference list of books and articles cited in the works. All are valid ways to gather additional information.

Evaluating, Revising, and Storing Search Results

Whether EBP team members conduct a search individually or with the help of a medical librarian, it is the searcher's responsibility to evaluate the results for relevance and quality. Keep in mind that to answer the clinical question thoroughly, a team's search strategies may need several revisions, and they should allow adequate time for these alterations. A good way to eliminate lower-quality literature in an initial review is to judge the resources using the following criteria (Johns Hopkins University—The Sheridan Libraries, 2010):

- *Who wrote it?* What is the author's affiliation, background, intent, or bias?

- *Who is the intended audience?* Is it intended for specialists, practitioners, the general public, or another targeted group?

- *What is the scope or coverage?* Is the resource meant to give a general overview, foundational introduction, detailed investigation, cutting-edge update, or some other level of detail?

- *Why was it written or published?* Is it meant to inform, explain, entertain, or persuade? Is it intended to be objective and neutral or controversial?

- *How current is it?* When was it published and last updated?

- *Where or by whom was it published?* Does this individual or group have a particular role or agenda? If relevant, what is the source of funding?

- *How is the information presented?* Are sources or evidence cited? Are there bibliographies, footnotes, or other specific citations?

- *How accurate is it?* Is there an evidence trail? Are related sources cited in order to triangulate information or claims?

When revising a search, consider these questions:

- *When was the last search conducted?* If the search is several years old, you need to consider changes that may have happened in the field that were missed by the previous search.

- *Have new terms been developed related to your search question?* Terms often change. Even controlled vocabulary like MeSH is updated annually. Make sure to search for new controlled vocabulary and new keywords.

- *Did the search include databases beyond the nursing literature?* Are there databases outside of nursing that are relevant to your question? Does your question branch into psychology or physical therapy? Were those databases searched previously?

- *Are the limits used in the first search still appropriate?* If an age range limit was used in the last search, is it still relevant? Were there restrictions on publication type or methodology that are no longer useful?

After a successful search strategy is created, teams or individuals should keep a record of the work. Often individuals research the same topic throughout their career, so saving search strategies assists in updating work without duplication of effort. Most databases have a feature that allows saving a search within the database; however, it is always a good idea to keep multiple copies of searches. Microsoft Word documents or emails are a great way to keep a record of work.

PubMed is an example of a database that allows multiple searches to be saved. *My NCBI*, a companion piece to PubMed, permits users to create an account, save searches, set alerts, and customize preferences. Search results can also be saved by exporting them into a citation management software program such as *EndNote, RefWorks, Zotero, Mendeley*, or *Papers*. Though some citation management programs are free, others need to be purchased; some may be provided for free by an organization. The function and capabilities of the various programs are similar.

After the citations are identified, the next step is to obtain the full text. If the full text is not available online, request the local library to obtain the information through the interlibrary loan service. This request may be free if the local library is affiliated with a university or institute, but it may require a fee if the request for resources is made from a public library.

Summary

This chapter illustrates how to use the PICO as a guide for literature searches. An essential component of EBP, the literature search is important to any research-and-publication activity because it enables researchers to acquire a better understanding of the topic and an awareness of relevant literature. Information specialists, such as medical librarians, can help with complex search strategies and information retrieval.

Ideally, an iterative search process is used and includes: examining indexed databases, using keywords in searches, studying the resulting articles, and, finally, refining the searches for optimal retrieval. The use of keywords, controlled vocabulary, Boolean operators, and limits plays an important role in finding the most relevant material for the practice problem. Alerting services are effective in helping researchers keep up-to-date with a research topic. Exploring and selecting from the wide array of published information can be a time-consuming task, so plan carefully so that you can carry out this work effectively.

References

Bramer, W. M., Giustini, D., & Kramer, B. M. R. (2016). Comparing the coverage, recall, and precision of searches for 120 systematic reviews in Embase, MEDLINE, and Google Scholar: A prospective study. *Systematic Reviews*, 5(39). doi: 10.1186/s13643-016-0215-7

Hartzell, T.A., Fineout-Overholt, E., Hofstetter, S., & Ponder, E. (2015). Finding relevant evidence to answer clinical questions. In B. M. Melnyk & E. Fineout-Overholt (Eds.), *Evidence-Based Practice in Nursing and Healthcare: A Guide to Best Practice* (3rd ed.) (pp. 40–73). Philadelphia, PA: Wolters Kluwer Health.

Johns Hopkins University—The Sheridan Libraries. (2010). *Expository writing: The research process: Evaluating sources*. Retrieved from http://guides.library.jhu.edu/content.php?pid=24792&sid=179624

Johnson, J. H. (2015). Evidence-based practice. In M. J. Smith, R. Carpenter, & J. J. Fitzpatrick (Eds.) *Encyclopedia of Nursing Education* (1st ed.). (pp. 144–146). New York, NY: Springer Publishing Company, LLC.

McCulley, C., & Jones, M. (2014). Fostering RN-to-BSN students' confidence in searching online for scholarly information on evidence-based practice. *The Journal of Continuing Education in Nursing, 45*(1), 22–27. doi: http://dx.doi.org/10.3928/00220124-20131223-01

6

Evidence Appraisal: Research

Most evidence-rating schemes recognize that the strongest evidence accumulates from scientific evidence, also referred to as research. Within the broad realm of research, studies vary in terms of the level, quality, and strength of evidence they provide. The level of evidence is determined by the type of research design; the quality of evidence is determined by critical appraisal of study methods for validity and reliability; and the strength of evidence is determined through synthesis of the level and quality of evidence. Practice recommendations based on sound scientific evidence have a greater likelihood of positively impacting patient outcomes (Melnyk & Newhouse, 2014).

This chapter provides:

- An overview of the various types of research evidence
- Information on appraising the level and quality of research evidence
- Tips for reading research evidence

Publications That Report Scientific Evidence

Research evidence can be broadly grouped into reports of single research studies (experimental, quasi-experimental, nonexperimental, qualitative designs) and summaries of multiple research studies (systematic reviews with or without meta-analysis or meta-synthesis). The level of research evidence for single studies is determined by the study design. For summaries of multiple studies, the level of evidence is based on the types of designs of the studies included in the summaries.

Most often, an evidence-based practice (EBP) team retrieves reports of primary research studies. *Primary* research comprises data that are collected to answer one or more research questions. Reviewers may also find *secondary* analyses that use data from primary studies to ask different questions. EBP teams need to recognize and appraise each evidence type and the relative strength it provides. A working knowledge of the strengths and limitations of the various types of research studies enables the nurse to judge the relative quality of evidence.

Summaries of Multiple Studies

Published reports of summaries of multiple research studies, also referred to as systematic reviews, can include quantitative, qualitative, or both types of research. This section describes systematic reviews (with or without meta-analysis or meta-synthesis—defined later in this discussion) as a source of evidence. Notable efforts include the Cochrane Collaboration (2016), an international nonprofit organization that produces and disseminates systematic reviews of healthcare interventions, and *Worldviews on Evidence-Based Nursing* (2016), a peer-reviewed journal developed by the Sigma Theta Tau International Honor Society of Nursing. A less prominent but growing effort focused on methods and processes involved in the synthesis of qualitative evidence has been undertaken by the Cochrane Qualitative and Implementation Methods Group. The *Cochrane Handbook for Systematic Reviews of Interventions* (Higgins & Green, 2015) includes a chapter providing guidance for using evidence from qualitative research to help explain, interpret, and apply the results of a Cochrane review.

Systematic Reviews

Systematic reviews summarize critically appraised research evidence (usually experimental and quasi-experimental studies) related to a specific question. Such reviews employ and document comprehensive search strategies and rigorous, transparent appraisal methods. Bias is minimized when a group of experts, rather than individuals, applies standardized methods to the review process. The Institute of Medicine (2011) appointed an expert committee to establish methodological standards for developing and reporting of all types of systematic reviews.

The Agency for Healthcare Research and Quality (AHRQ) awards 5-year contracts to North American institutions to serve as Evidence-based Practice Centers (EPCs). EPCs review scientific literature on clinical, behavioral, organizational, and financial topics to produce evidence reports and technology assessments (EPC Evidence-Based Reports, 2016). Additionally, EPCs conduct research on systematic review methodology. A *systematic review* is interchangeable with an *evidence report*.

Systematic reviews use *meta-analysis* or *meta-synthesis* to analyze the combined results of multiple research studies. Systematic reviews of quantitative studies are referred to as *meta-analyses*. Meta-analysis provides a more precise estimate of the effects of healthcare interventions than those derived from individual studies included in the review by providing a common metric, which is called an effect size (Polit & Beck, 2017). Through use of statistical methods, meta-analysis aids in understanding not only the existence of a relationship between study variables but also an estimate of the magnitude of the relationships across studies (Polit & Beck, 2017). Meta-analyses that include only randomized controlled trials (RCTs) are Level I evidence. Meta-analyses that contain quasi-experimental studies are categorized at a lower level of evidence.

When a systematic review summarizes the results of independent qualitative studies, it is referred to as a *meta-synthesis*. Meta-synthesis combines the results from a number of qualitative studies to arrive at a deeper understanding of the phenomenon under review and produces a broader interpretation than can be gained from a single qualitative study.

Systematic reviews differ from more traditional narrative literature reviews. Narrative reviews often contain references to research studies but do not critically appraise, evaluate, and summarize the relative merits of the included studies. True systematic reviews address both the strengths and limitations of each study included in the review. Readers should not differentiate between a systematic review and a narrative literature review based solely on the title of the article. At times, the title will state that the article presents a literature review when it is in fact a systematic review or state that the article is a systematic review when it is a literature review. EBP teams generally consider themselves lucky when they uncover well-executed systematic reviews that include summative research techniques that apply to the practice question of interest. Table 6.1 outlines the defining features of systematic reviews and reviews that include meta-analysis or meta-synthesis.

Table 6.1   Defining Features of Summative Research Techniques

Summative Evidence	Description	Defining Features
Systematic review	Review of research evidence related to a specific clinical question	▪ Employs comprehensive, reproducible search strategies and rigorous appraisal methods ▪ Can include experimental and non-experimental research studies
Meta-analysis	Research technique that synthesizes and analyzes quantitative scientific evidence	▪ Uses statistical procedures to combine results from independent primary studies ▪ Usually includes experimental and/or quasi-experimental studies ▪ Estimates overall effect size of a specific intervention or variable on a defined outcome
Meta-synthesis	Research technique that synthesizes and analyzes qualitative scientific evidence	▪ Limited to qualitative studies ▪ Identification of key metaphors and concepts ▪ Interprets and translates findings

Meta-Analysis

Meta-analysis offers the advantage of objectivity because the decisions made by the study reviewers are explicit, and the integration of studies uses statistics applied to the data set (Polit & Beck, 2017). By combining the results of multiple studies in a meta-analysis, the number of study participants from each individual study are combined. This increases the statistical power and the probability of detecting a true relationship between the independent and dependent variables (Polit & Beck, 2017). As mentioned earlier, the common metric called *effect size* (ES), a measure of the strength of the relationship between two variables, is developed for each of the primary studies. A positive ES indicates a positive relationship (as one variable increases, the second variable increases); a negative ES indicates a negative relationship (as one variable increases or decreases, the second variable moves in the opposite direction). By combining results across a number of smaller studies, the researcher can increase the power, or the probability, of detecting a true relationship between the intervention and the outcomes of the intervention (Polit & Beck, 2017). When combining studies for meta-analysis, the researcher can statistically analyze only those interventions (independent variables) and outcomes (dependent variables) that the studies have in common. The results of the meta-analysis are often displayed in a forest plot (see Figure 6.1). A *forest plot*, which is a graphical representation of a meta-analysis, is usually accompanied by a table listing references (author and date) of the studies included in the meta-analysis and the statistical results (Centre for Evidence-Based Intervention, n.d.).

An *overall summary statistic* combines and averages ESs across studies. An investigator should describe the method that determined the ES and should help the reader interpret the statistic. Cohen's (1988) methodology for determining ESs includes the following strength of correlation ratings: trivial (ES = 0.01–0.09), low to moderate (0.10–0.29), moderate to substantial (0.30–0.49), substantial to very strong (0.50–0.69), very strong (0.70–0.89), and almost perfect (0.90–0.99).

Example: Meta-Analysis

Nam, Janson, Stotts, Chesla, & Kroon (2012) conducted a systematic review of randomized controlled trials to examine the effect of culturally tailored diabetes education in ethnic minorities with Type 2 diabetes. They applied statistics to the pooled results of 12 RCTs that had sufficient data to include in a meta-analysis. The independent variable was diabetes educational interventions performed in ethnic minority groups with Type 2 diabetes, and the dependent variable was glycemic control measured by HbA1c levels.

Study or Subgroup	Treatment n/N	Control n/N		Risk Ration (95% CI)
Gamsu 1989	15/131	22/137		0.71 [0.39-1.31]
Garite 1992	12/36	12/41		1.14 [0.59-2.21]
Kari 1994	5/95	6/94		0.82 [0.26-2.61]
Liggins 1972a	108/601	122/617		0.91 [0.72-1.15]
Parsons 1988	0/23	1/22		0.32 [0.01-7.45]
Qublan 2001	21/72	41/67		0.48 [0.32-0.72]
Schutte 1980	6/65	12/58		0.45 [0.18-1.11]
Taeusch 1979	10/56	12/71		1.06 [0.49-2.27]
Subtotal (95% CI)	**1813**	**1814**		**0.77 [0.67-0.89]**

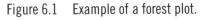

0.2   0.5   1.0   2.0   5.0

Figure 6.1   Example of a forest plot.

Image adapted from Table 4, Roberts & Dalziel, 2006

Meta-Synthesis

In contrast to numbers-based quantitative research, qualitative research is text-based. Qualitative researchers collect rich narrative materials; integration of these data results in a grand narrative or interpretative translation (Polit & Beck,

2017). Meta-synthesis is thought of as the qualitative counterpart to meta-analysis and involves interpreting data rather than aggregating data or producing a summary statistic (Polit & Beck, 2017). In meta-synthesis, researchers make systematic decisions on study inclusion criteria and evaluate the study quality. Both meta-analyses and meta-syntheses use rigorous scientific techniques.

A number of different types of meta-synthesis methods exist. One commonly used method is meta-ethnography (Noblit & Hare, 1988). *Meta-ethnography*, which has its origins in the field of education, involves seven phases that focus on the translation and interpretation of findings (Polit & Beck, 2017). Other meta-synthesis methods include *qualitative meta-summary, critical interpretive synthesis, grounded formal theory, thematic synthesis*, and *meta-study* (Polit & Beck, 2017). For nurses who lack experience and expertise in critiquing qualitative studies, meta-syntheses are quite helpful because they aid in not only assessing the rigor of individual studies but also interpreting findings.

Example: Meta-Synthesis

Flores, Leblanc, and Barroso (2016) conducted a meta-synthesis to understand the factors that influence how a person with human immunodeficiency virus (HIV) is linked and retained in care. They synthesized 69 studies that included either qualitative research studies or the qualitative results from mixed-methods studies. The meta-synthesis included 2,263 HIV-positive participants and 994 healthcare providers, family members, or community members. Researchers found three themes, or influences, for how persons with HIV interact with the care system: 1) the interpersonal stream that includes psychological state upon diagnosis and informational challenges; 2) the social stream that includes societal experiences and provider interaction; and 3) the cultural-attitudinal stream including life demands, quality-of-care experiences, and other structural barriers. The findings from this meta-synthesis suggest that there are reasons, other than individual level factors, that link and retain persons with HIV in care. Flores et al. suggested that changes are needed to address the social and cultural-attitudinal influences.

Individual Research Studies

The EBP team begins its evidence search in the hope of finding the highest level of scientific evidence available on the topic of interest. Table 6.2 outlines the distinctive features of the various types of research designs and evidence the team may uncover.

Table 6.2   Research Designs, Distinctive Features, and Examples

Research Design	Distinctive Features	Examples
Experimental	<ul><li>An intervention</li><li>Control</li><li>Random assignment to the intervention or control group</li><li>Manipulation of one variable</li></ul>	<ul><li>Randomized controlled trial</li></ul>
Quasi-experimental	<ul><li>An intervention</li><li>Lacks either a control group or random assignment to the intervention group</li></ul>	<ul><li>Nonequivalent control (comparison) group: posttest only or pretest–posttest</li><li>One group: posttest only or pretest–posttest</li><li>Time series</li><li>Untreated control, repeated measures</li><li>Repeated treatment where subjects serve as their own controls</li><li>Crossover design</li></ul>

Research Design	Distinctive Features	Examples
Nonexperimental (quantitative)	■ May have an intervention ■ No random assignment to group(s) ■ No control group	■ Descriptive ■ Predictive ■ Explanatory ■ Time-dimensional
Qualitative	■ No randomization ■ No manipulation ■ Little control of the natural environment	■ Basic qualitative descriptive ■ Ethnography ■ Grounded theory ■ Phenomenology ■ Narrative inquiry ■ Case study
Mixed methods	■ Includes both quantitative and qualitative elements ■ Combination of quantitative and qualitative elements may provide more than either by itself	■ Convergent parallel ■ Explanatory sequential ■ Exploratory sequential ■ Multiphasic

Experimental Studies

Experimental studies, or RCTs, use the traditional scientific method. The investigator obtains verifiable, objective, research-based knowledge by observing or measuring in a manner such that resulting evidence is reproducible. Types of experimental designs that an EBP team may encounter include pretest–posttest control group (the original, most widely used experimental design); posttest only; randomized block; wait-list control group (delay of intervention design); and crossover/repeated measures (Polit & Beck, 2017).

A true experimental study has three distinctive features: *randomization, control,* and *manipulation*. *Randomization* occurs when the researcher assigns subjects to a control or experimental group randomly, similar to the roll of dice. This ensures that each potential subject who meets inclusion criteria has the same probability of selection for the experiment. That is, people in the experimental group and in the control group generally will be identical, except for the introduction of the experimental intervention or treatment. This is important because subjects who take part in an experiment serve as representatives of the population that may possibly benefit from the intervention.

Manipulation occurs when the researcher implements an intervention with at least some of the subjects. In experimental research, an intervention is applied to some subjects (the *experimental group*) and withheld from others (the *control group*). The aspect that the researcher is trying to influence is the *dependent variable* (e.g., the experience of low back pain). The experimental intervention is the *independent variable,* or the action the researcher will take (e.g., application of low-level heat therapy) to try to change the dependent variable.

Control usually refers to the introduction of a control or comparison group, such as a group of subjects to which the experimental intervention is *not* applied. The goal is to compare the effect of no intervention on the dependent variable in the control group against the effect of the experimental intervention on the dependent variable in the experimental group. Placebos, which may be given to subjects in the control group, are used as a pseudo-intervention because they are assumed by researchers to have no therapeutic value (Polit & Beck, 2017). When placebos are used, they control for nonintervention effects such as attention being paid to subjects and subjects' expectations of benefits and harms.

Example: Experimental Randomized Controlled Trial

Kiecolt-Glaser et al. (2014) reported on an experimental study investigating yoga's impact on inflammation, mood, and fatigue in breast cancer survivors. Following randomization, participants were assigned to either 12 weeks of 90-minute hatha yoga classes or a wait-list control. Participants assigned to wait-list control were told to continue usual activities and refrain from beginning any yoga practice. After final study assessment, wait-list controls were offered the yoga classes.

Quasi-Experimental Studies

Quasi-experimental studies are similar to experimental studies in that they try to show that an intervention causes a particular outcome. These designs are used when it is not possible to meet two of the three requirements for an experimental study. Quasi-experimental studies always include manipulation of the independent variable. They differ from experimental studies because it is not possible to have either a control group or random assignment of subjects. For example, an investigator can assign the intervention (manipulation) to one of two groups (e.g., two medical units), with one serving as the intervention group and one serving as the control group. The investigator cannot randomly assign participants to the units.

In cases where a particular intervention is effective, withholding that intervention would be unethical. In the same vein, it would not be practical to perform a study that requires more human, financial, and material resources than are available. At times, neither patients nor geographical locations can be randomized. Consider the investigator who wants to study the effect of bed-exit alarms on patient falls. It would not be easy to randomize the use of bed-exit alarms to individual patient rooms or to individual patients. Nursing staff likely would not agree to deactivate bed-exit alarms on at-risk patients whose beds are equipped with this safety feature. Quasi-experimental designs that an EBP team may uncover during the course of its search include nonequivalent control (comparison) group posttest only and nonequivalent control (comparison) group pretest–posttest. The term *nonequivalent* means not only that assignment is nonrandom but also that the researcher does not control assignment to groups. This design is most often used when doing research with intact groups. Hence, groups may be different on important variables such as health status or demographics, and group differences may affect outcomes. Other quasi-experimental research study designs are not included in this chapter. EBP team members should refer to a research text when they encounter any unfamiliar study designs.

Examples: Quasi-Experimental Studies

Labrague and McEnroe-Petitte (2014) conducted a study to determine the influence of music on anxiety levels and physiologic parameters in women undergoing gynecologic surgery. The study used a pretest and posttest experimental design with nonrandom assignment to control group (nonmusic group) or experimental group (music group). The study is quasi-experimental rather than purely experimental; although it included a music intervention *(manipulation)* and no music *(control),* the subjects were not randomly assigned to each group.

Nonexperimental Studies

Similar to experimental research designs, nonexperimental research designs are the blueprint for all aspects needed to carry out the study—overall for the collection, measurement, and analysis of data. When reviewing evidence related to healthcare questions, particularly inquiries of interest to nursing, EBP teams will often find studies of naturally occurring phenomena (groups, treatments, and individuals). These studies are considered nonexperimental or observational in design. The studies may or may not introduce an intervention. Subjects are not randomly assigned to different groups, variables are not manipulated, and the investigator is not always able to control aspects of the environment.

Quantitative nonexperimental studies can be classified by research purpose and by time dimension (Belli, 2009). Three categories classified by purpose, or intent, are *descriptive, predictive,* and *explanatory.* Categories classified by time are *prospective, longitudinal,* and *retrospective.*

Descriptive Designs

The intent of purely *descriptive* designs, as the name implies, is to *describe* or identify situations or characteristics of phenomena. Basic questions asked in descriptive research are: What are the quantifiable values of particular variables for a given set of subjects? How widespread is a phenomenon? Variables are not manipulated, and no attempt is made to determine that a particular intervention or characteristic is related to or causes a specific occurrence to happen.

The investigators seek to provide the *who, what, where, when,* and *how* of particular persons, places, or things. An attempt is made to describe the answers to these questions in precisely measured terms. Statistical analysis is generally limited to frequencies and averages. Common types of descriptive designs include *univariate descriptive, descriptive comparative, descriptive correlational,* and *epidemiologic descriptive* studies (prevalence and incidence). Table 6.3 on page 112 outlines the features of descriptive designs and purpose.

Univariate descriptive studies, which often use exploratory or survey designs, aim to describe the frequency of a behavior or an occurrence. Univariate descriptive studies are "not necessarily focused on only one variable …there are multiple variables …but the primary purpose is to describe the status of each and not to relate them to one another" (Polit & Beck, 2017). Exploratory and survey designs are common in nursing and healthcare. When little knowledge about the phenomenon of interest exists, these designs offer the greatest degree of flexibility. Though new information is learned, the direction of the exploration may change. With exploratory designs, the investigator does not know enough about a phenomenon to identify variables of interest completely. Variables are observed as they happen; there is no researcher control. When investigators know enough about a particular phenomenon and can identify specific variables of interest, a descriptive survey design more fully describes the phenomenon. Questionnaire (survey) or interview techniques assess the variables of interest.

> **Example: Nonexperimental Descriptive Survey Design**
>
> Bourgault et al. (2014) conducted a national online survey of critical-care nurses to examine factors that influence the adoption of the American Association of Critical-Care Nurses practice alert on the verification of feeding tube placement and the adoption of four clinical practices recommended in the guideline. There was no intervention, researcher control, or randomization; the intent was to describe existing practices.

Descriptive comparative designs look at and describe differences in variables between or among two or more groups. No attempt is made to determine causality. Generally, descriptive statistics, such as frequency distributions and measures of central tendency (mean, median, and mode), are used to summarize these differences.

Example: Nonexperimental Descriptive Comparative Design

Stickney, Ziniel, Brett, & Truog (2014) used a cross-sectional survey to compare parental and healthcare providers' attitudes and experiences of family participation during unit rounds in a tertiary pediatric ICU. Parents and healthcare provider questionnaires were developed in parallel to allow for direct comparison of their perceptions of selected dimensions of rounds. Researchers administered the questionnaires *(surveys)* to a convenience sample *(nonrandom)* of parents and healthcare providers and described differences in responses between the two groups.

Descriptive correlational designs seek to describe relationships among variables. Again, no attempt is made to understand causal relationships. The investigator gathers information on at least two variables and conducts a statistical correlation analysis between the two variables of interest to obtain a *correlation coefficient*—a number ranging from –1 to 1. The correlation coefficient tells the *direction* of the association between the two variables. If the correlation coefficient is between 0 and 1, the correlation is positive: As one variable of interest increases, so does the second variable. A negative correlation is depicted by correlation coefficients between –1 and 0: As one variable increases, the other variable decreases. The correlation coefficient also tells the reader the strength or *magnitude* of the correlation—that is, the closer this coefficient is to 1 (if positive) or –1 (if negative), the stronger the association between the two variables.

Example: Nonexperimental Descriptive Correlational Design

Dabney and Kalisch (2015) examined patient reports of missed care and levels of nurse staffing. The researchers used Pearson Correlation Coefficients to describe the relationship between missed care (basic care, communication, timeliness) and staffing levels (RN hours per patient day [HPPD], Nursing HPPD, RN skill mix). Lack of timeliness was negatively associated with total Nursing HPPD ($r = -0.09$), RNHPPD ($r = -0.14$) and RN skill mix ($r = -0.13$).

Prevalence and incidence studies are descriptive designs frequently used by epidemiological researchers (Polit & Beck, 2017). The aim of prevalence studies is to determine the proportion of a population that has a particular condition at a specific point in time (known as *prevalence* or *point prevalence*). This provides researchers with a useful metric to better understand the burden of a specific disease in the community. Incidence studies seek to determine the frequency of new cases (or *incidence rate*) and are useful in understanding risk for disease development.

Example: Nonexperimental Epidemiological Descriptive Designs

An interdisciplinary research team (Dybitz, Thompson, Molotsky, & Stuart, 2011) studied the prevalence of diabetes and the burden of comorbid conditions in elderly nursing home residents. Prevalence of diabetes was determined by laboratory values recorded in the medical record over a 12-month period, documented medical-chart diagnosis of diabetes, and evidence of medications prescribed for diabetes in a prescription claims database. They found a diabetes prevalence of 32.8% of residents from a national sample of 250 skilled nursing facilities and characterized the disease burden of diabetes in these settings.

Roberts (2010) conducted electronic chart reviews of hospitalized children in a midsize urban hospital over a 2-week period to determine the incidence of parental/guardian absence in the previous 24 hours. The researchers were interested in understanding the risk for unaccompanied pediatric patients in a culture that promotes patient-family centered care.

Predictive Designs

Predictive designs seek to *predict* relationships. Two basic questions are asked in predictive research: "If phenomenon X occurs, will phenomenon Y follow? If we introduce an intervention, will a particular outcome follow?" Predictive designs range from simple predictive correlational studies that look at whether a single variable predicts a particular outcome to more complex predictive designs that use multiple or logistic regression to examine whether several variables predict a particular outcome.

Example: Nonexperimental Predictive Correlational Design

Mazanec, Daly, Douglas, and Musil (2011) used a predictive correlational design to examine the role of cognitive appraisal in predicting post-radiation treatment psychological adjustment in women with various forms of cancer. The research team prospectively examined the relationship between cognitive appraisal and psychological adjustment (outcome variable).

Table 6.3   Descriptive Designs and Purpose

Title	Definition/Purpose	Notes
Univariate descriptive studies	Explain the frequency of a behavior or an occurrence.	Questionnaires, surveys.
Descriptive comparative designs	List differences between two or more groups on one or more independent variables to find out why the variables are different.	Groups that are similar in some but differ in other respects; the differences become the focus of examination.
Descriptive correlational designs	Describe relationships among variables by statistical analysis.	As one relationship varies, the other varies in the same or opposite direction; does not determine whether one variable causes another.
Prevalence studies	Determine the proportion of a population that has a particular condition at a specific point in time.	Useful to compare prevalence of disease in different populations or to examine trends in disease severity over time.
Incidence studies	Determine the frequency (or incidence rate) of new cases.	Useful in understanding risk for disease development.
Predictive designs	Predict future relationships or outcomes based on patterns within a set of variables.	Applies statistical methods and/ or data mining techniques, without preconceived theoretical constructs.

Time-Dimensional Designs

Time-dimensional designs answer questions such as, "Were the data for the dependent and independent variables collected at a single point in time, or across a certain period, or did data already exist?" An EBP team should understand the concepts of retrospective, prospective, and longitudinal with respect to examining a phenomenon over time. In *retrospective* studies, the investigator looks at proposed causes, and the effects that have already happened, to learn from the past. In contrast, *prospective* studies examine causes that may have occurred in the past and then look forward in time to observe the presumed effects. *Longitudinal* studies look at changes in the same subjects over a long period. The basic question asked in longitudinal (present) and prospective (future) research is, "What are the differences in a variable or variables over time, going from the present to the future?" The basic question in retrospective studies is, "What differences in a variable or variables existed in the past that may explain present differences in these variables?"

Three common types of descriptive or observational studies that have a time component are *case-control, cohort,* and *cross-sectional*. Because unfamiliar terminology can divert the reviewer's attention from review of a study, an understanding of these terms should minimize confusion. Table 6.4 outlines time-dimensional designs and purposes.

Case-control studies, which are used in epidemiologic research, examine possible relationships between exposure and disease occurrence. "The hallmark of the case control study is that it begins with people with the disease (cases) and compares them to people without the disease (controls)" (Gordis, 2009, p. 179). The basic question asked in case-control studies is, "Is there a relationship between being exposed to particular phenomena and contracting a specific disease?" Case-control studies compare the proportion of cases that have a particular condition or outcome with the proportion of cases that do not have the condition or outcome (Lu, 2009). This proportion is expressed as an odds ratio, which is a way of comparing whether the probability of a certain condition or outcome occurring is the same as the probability of the condition or outcome not occurring. An illustration of a case-control study (see Figure 6.2) considers body mass index (BMI) as a determinant of obesity in the population of interest.

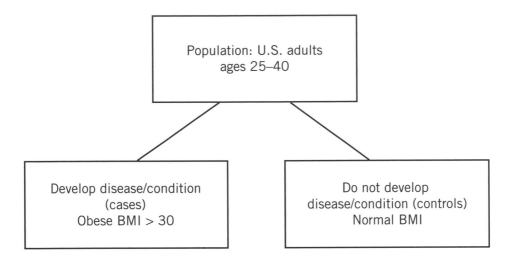

Figure 6.2   Illustration of a case-control study.

Example: Nonexperimental Descriptive Case-Control Design

Early detection of signs of sepsis can decrease mortality. Back, Jin, Jin, & Lee (2016) used data mining techniques analyzing electronic health records (EHRs) to identify predictors of sepsis. The study used a retrospective 1:4 case control review. Study patients with sepsis were the case group, and patients without sepsis were the control group. The team used EHR data for a 4-year period at the study hospital to identify seven predictors of sepsis and develop a sepsis risk scoring algorithm.

Cohort studies look at a particular subset of a population from which different samples are taken at various points in time. These types of observational studies can be retrospective, in which both the exposure and the outcome of interest has already occurred, or prospective, in which the patients who have been exposed to the condition of interest are observed to determine the occurrence of the outcome of interest (Lu, 2009). Cohort studies that are prospective may require a long-term follow-up period until the outcome event has occurred (Gordis, 2009). The risk factor of smoking in the population is used to illustrate a prospective cohort study (see Figure 6.3):

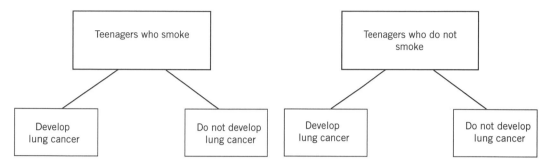

Figure 6.3   Illustration of a prospective cohort study.

Example: Nonexperimental Descriptive Cohort Design

A group of researchers in the United Kingdom used Clinical Practice Research Datalink files from 2004 to 2014 to study the probability of an obese person attaining normal body weight or a 5% reduction in body weight. The study included 76,704 obese men and 99,701 obese women. In examining this cohort, the probability of attaining normal weight or maintaining weight loss was low. The annual probability of attaining normal weight was 1 in 210 for men and 1 in 124 for obese women, not including the morbidly obese. The researchers concluded that obesity treatment programs grounded in community-based weight management programs may be ineffective (Fildes et al., 2015).

Cross-sectional studies involve the collection of data at one particular point in time. These studies collect a representative sample and classify by outcome and risk factor simultaneously. The basic question asked in cross-sectional research is, "What are the characteristics of a population at a single point in time?" In epidemiology, the researcher starts with a defined population and gathers data on the presence or absence of exposure and the presence or absence of disease for each individual at a particular point. Prevalence studies employ epidemiological cross-sectional designs. In other types of studies using a cross-sectional design, the researcher looks at variables in a population at a single point.

Example: Nonexperimental Descriptive Cross-Sectional Design

Finnish researchers used a descriptive cross-sectional design to conduct a national survey at four Finnish university hospitals to understand the differences in RNs' EBP competencies and job-related nurse outcomes in non-Magnet university hospitals. A convenience sample of 943 practice nurses responded. Findings included that nurses' EBP beliefs were favorable, and that nurses were satisfied with their jobs; however, they lacked the EBP knowledge required for integrating best evidence into clinical care (Saunders & Vehviläinen-Julkunen, 2016).

Table 6.4   Time-Dimensional Designs, Purposes, and Examples

Title	Purpose	Notes
Case-control studies	Compares the proportion of cases that have a particular condition or outcome with the proportion of cases that do not have the condition	Examines possible relationships between exposure and disease occurrence and is expressed as an odds ratio
Cohort studies	Investigates the causes of disease, establishing links between risk factors and health outcomes	Observational studies that can be retrospective or prospective studies
Cross-sectional studies	Collects data at one particular point in time	

Qualitative Designs

Qualitative designs have their roots in sociology and are often used to answer the "how" or "why" research questions. The purpose of qualitative research is to explore, discover, or describe. In contrast to quantitative research, qualitative researchers are often active participants in research activities, acknowledging their personal values and bringing their own experience to the study. Qualitative research, which is the best way to understand phenomena deeply and in detail, is useful when exploring complex situations or areas where little is known.

Within qualitative design, a researcher may use one of many methods to answer the research question. Each methodology has its own purpose, and data are often collected and analyzed in quite different ways. Examples of qualitative methods are *basic qualitative descriptive, ethnography, grounded theory, phenomenology, narrative inquiry,* and *case study* (see Table 6.5).

Basic qualitative descriptive designs are surface descriptions of events or experiences, and they involve limited interpretation by the researcher (Sandelowski, 2000). This methodology often includes characteristics from the other qualitative methodologies, such as the use of constant comparison from grounded theory, and content analysis is frequently used for data analysis (Sandelowski, 2000). Basic qualitative descriptive studies produce findings that are simple representations of the data likely to be agreed on by researchers and participants (Sandelowski, 2000).

Example: Basic Qualitative Descriptive Design

Shafir et al. (2016) conducted a basic qualitative descriptive study in order to understand what homebound older adults and their caregivers described as quality care. The researchers developed their interview guide from a literature review and included questions addressing the Department of Health and Human Services Multiple Chronic Conditions key measurement concepts. The team also used these key measurement concepts as the framework for their analysis. Findings from the study included five themes related to quality care; the researchers suggest changes to the way health was delivered in order to meet what they found to be quality care.

Ethnography, with roots in anthropology, describes and analyzes characteristics of the ways of life of cultures or subcultures and is of growing interest to nurses who seek to provide culturally competent care (de Chesnay, 2014). The researcher is required to gain entry into the culture being studied, often spending extended periods observing the behaviors of people in the culture (de Chesnay, 2014). Researchers immerse themselves in the culture and keep extensive field notes or reflexive journals, which are categorized and analyzed to discover major themes.

Example: Qualitative Ethnography Design

The ethnographic study of Curtis and Northcott (2016) explored how children, parents, and nurses in a pediatric hospital experienced family-centered care. The researchers were interested in how the spaces within the hospital—particularly, single and shared rooms—affected family-centered care. The 2-phase study included observations (Phase 1) within four pediatric units and interviews and focus groups (Phase 2) with children, parents, and nurses or support staff. Curtis and Northcott found two themes from analysis—role expectations and family-nurse interactions—and concluded that the spaces within the hospital change how family-centered care occurs.

Grounded theory designs seek to examine the basic social and psychological problems/concerns that characterize real-world phenomena and to identify the process used to resolve these problems/concerns (Polit & Beck, 2017). In this type of qualitative research design, the researcher simultaneously collects and analyzes data to generate concepts and integrate these concepts into a data-grounded theory that explains a process (Birks & Mills, 2015). Data analysis is done by way of coding.

Example: Qualitative Grounded Theory Design

Hyatt, Davis, and Barroso (2015) used grounded theory to understand the process by which soldiers returning from Iraq and Afghanistan with mild traumatic brain injury (mTBI) reintegrated into their family life. The researchers theoretically selected their sample in order to continuously compare and test the themes as they emerged from the data from previous participants. After interviewing nine soldiers with mTBI and their spouses, Hyatt, Davis, and Barroso concluded that reintegrating into family life following mTBI was "finding a new normal." The researchers recommend future interventions to assist family adjustment to a new normal and management of mismatched expectations.

Phenomenology originates in philosophy and examines an experience as people live it rather than as they conceptualize it. Phenomenological research seeks to understand what an experience means and what the lived experience of a person is. The researcher collects data primarily by way of in-depth conversations, and sample sizes are often small (Polit & Beck, 2017). Phenomenology includes descriptive phenomenology and interpretive phenomenology, two methods that differ in their emphasis on either describing or interpreting and understanding an experience (Polit & Beck, 2017).

Example: Qualitative Phenomenology Design

MacWilliams, Hughes, Aston, Field, and Wight Moffatt (2016) used interpretive phenomenology to describe what women who are having a miscarriage experience when they arrive at the emergency department. The study included interviews with eight women, and findings described that all participants experienced a loss and emotional burden following miscarriage. Participants felt that their experiences were different from others seeking care in the emergency department because they had experienced loss, and were not ill. The researchers concluded that nurses in the emergency department caring for women experiencing miscarriage acknowledge the loss and emotions the women may feel and prepare the women for the experiences they may have after discharge from the emergency department.

Narrative inquiry, or narrative analysis, is a methodology in qualitative research where the researcher examines the story a participant tells, and it may be an appropriate methodology for researching sensitive topics. Although, like phenomenology, it has roots in philosophy, narrative inquiry acknowledges the researcher's subjectivity, compared to the objective nature of phenomenology (Chunfeng Wang & Geale, 2015). Narrative inquiry is dependent on the researcher-participant relationship, and the trust between the two allows the researcher to uncover details in the participant's story (Chunfeng Wang & Geale, 2015).

Example: Qualitative Narrative Inquiry Design

Reed, Rowe, and Barnes (2015) used narrative inquiry to explore midwifery practice during an uncomplicated birth. The research included in-depth interviews with ten midwives and ten mothers who were asked to tell their stories. Instead of being asked interview questions, the midwives were asked to tell a story about a birth and what they had done, and the mothers were asked to tell their birth stories. The researchers found two themes in the participants' stories—rites of passage and rites of protection—and concluded that birth is a liminal state within a ritual and that the midwife was the ritual companion.

Qualitative case study methodology is an in-depth, comprehensive study of a case (Stake, 1995). A case may best be understood as a person or a group of people about which the researcher wants to learn more (Stake, 1995). For example, a case could consist of a single patient on a unit, but it could also consist of all patients on the unit. A case does not have to be a person and may instead be a program or a system; however, the researcher must make clear the definition of the case (Stake, 1995). Case study research often describes experiences and may be single-case or multiple-case designs (Stake, 1995).

Example: Qualitative Case Study Design

Mills, Chamberlain-Salaun, Harrison, Yates, and O'Shea (2016) conducted a single-case research study with early career registered nurses (ECRNs) in order to describe and explain the ECRNs' experiences during their first five years of practice. This study included interviews and focus groups with ECRNs. The study team was interested in understanding the experience of ECRNs to improve retention and reduce turnover and found six themes related to retention: 1) well-planned, supported, and structured transition periods; 2) consideration of rotation through different areas with a 6-month minimum for skills development; 3) empowering decision-making; 4) placement opportunities and choice in decisions of where to work; 5) career advice and support that considers ECRNs' personalities and skills; and 6) encouragement to reflect on career choices.

Table 6.5   Qualitative Designs, Source, and Focus

Type	Source	Focus
Basic qualitative descriptive	Includes characteristics from the other qualitative methodologies, such as the use of constant comparison from grounded theory	Surfaces descriptions of events or experiences and involves limited interpretation by the researcher
Ethnography	Anthropology	Describes and analyzes characteristics of the ways of life of cultures or subcultures

Type	Source	Focus
Grounded theory	Sociology, psychology	Examines the basic social and psychological problems/concerns that characterize real-world phenomena
Phenomenology	Philosophy	Examines the lived experience of the person
Narrative inquiry	Philosophy	Examines the story a participant tells
Case study		Describes an in-depth, comprehensive study of a case

Mixed-Methods Research

Because qualitative and quantitative research designs are complementary, many studies use a combination of both. Mixed-methods research often provides a more complete understanding than either quantitative or qualitative methodology used independently. As with quantitative and qualitative methods, there are different designs within mixed methods. The most common mixed-method designs used in nursing research are *convergent parallel, explanatory sequential, exploratory sequential,* and *multiphasic* (see Table 6.6 on page 124) (Beck & Harrison, 2016).

Convergent parallel is a mixed-method research design in which the quantitative and qualitative data are collected concurrently and both types of data are prioritized equally. Data are analyzed independently and then merged to provide a more complete understanding of the data (Creswell, 2014).

> **Example: Convergent Parallel Design**
>
> LaFond, Van Hulle Vincent, Oosterhouse, and Wilkie (2016) used a convergent parallel design to evaluate nurses' beliefs regarding pain in critically ill children. Registered nurses working at least 20 hours a week for the past year in a pediatric intensive care unit (PICU) completed the Pain Beliefs and Practices Questionnaire (PBPQ) and participated in semistructured interviews after viewing patient-scenario vignettes. Data collection occurred concurrently, and the research team analyzed both the PBPQ results and qualitative themes for points of convergence and divergence. Results from the study indicated that PICU nurses were knowledgeable about effective pain-management practices but needed additional information on pharmacokinetics.

Explanatory sequential designs are sequential designs with quantitative data collected in the initial phase, followed by qualitative data (Polit & Beck, 2017). These are basic questions for explanatory research: "What does a particular phenomenon look like? Does a particular theory explain the phenomenon of interest?"

> **Example: Explanatory Sequential Design**
>
> McConnell and Moroney (2015) conducted an explanatory sequential mixed-methods study in order to identify the barriers to involving relatives in patient care in the intensive care unit (ICU). The study team collected data from 70 critical-care nurses first using an online questionnaire. Results from the quantitative phase were used to inform the questions for the semistructured interviews. The study identified several barriers to involving relatives in care of the ICU patient: factors related to 1) the ICU patient, 2) the ICU relative, 3) the critical-care nurse, and 4) the intensive care environment.

Exploratory sequential designs begin with an exploratory qualitative phase of data collection and analysis followed by the quantitative phase. This design is often used when the qualitative findings need to be tested or generalized (Creswell, 2014). Exploratory sequential designs are well suited for studies related to theory development or instrument development.

> ### Example: Exploratory Sequential Design
>
> Al-Yateem (2013) aimed to develop guidelines to transition young adults from child to adult cystic fibrosis care. This study used an exploratory sequential design with two phases: the first, qualitative phase with focus groups of healthcare providers and the second, quantitative phase with a questionnaire. Findings from the focus groups yielded five themes and four categories. These findings were then used to develop the questionnaire that was completed by 171 healthcare providers and young adults with cystic fibrosis. Results from the survey were used to validate the guidelines, and 36 relevant and feasible guidelines from six categories for transitioning care were developed. Al-Yateem concluded that young adults' transition to adult cystic fibrosis care is addressed through assessment, planning, and continuous evaluation of care, provision of information, promotion of independence, and healthcare provider training.

Multiphasic, or multiphase, design is often used for program development and evaluation (Creswell, 2014). This type of design involves both qualitative and quantitative methods that are conducted in more than two phases. Data are collected and analyzed in phases, and each subsequent phase is informed by the results from the prior phase.

> ### Example: Multiphasic Design
>
> Sangster-Gormey, Griffith, Schreiber, and Borycki (2015) conducted a multiphase mixed-methods study to evaluate nurse practitioner (NP) integration in Canada. The study, conducted over three years, began with Phase 1, a quantitative survey of NPs. The researchers then added focus groups with NPs and chief nursing officers during the first year (Phase 2). Phase 2 also included surveys of patients and NPs' coworkers, as well as interviews and focus groups with NPs who had completed the survey in Phase 1. During Phase 3, the survey was administered to NPs and the results were compared to Phase 1. Researchers also used case studies of NPs to collect qualitative data during Phase 4. The study concluded with individual patient interviews to explore the patient perspective of NP care. This complex study allowed Sangster-Gormey et al. to comprehensively evaluate the integration of NPs and included perspectives of NPs, other healthcare professionals, and patients.

Table 6.6   Mixed-Methods Designs, Purpose, and Notes

Title	Purpose	Notes
Convergent parallel	Analyzes data independently and then merges data for interpretation	Design in which the quantitative and qualitative data are collected concurrently and both types of data are prioritized equally
Explanatory sequential	Used when quantitative findings are explained and interpreted with the assistance of qualitative data	Sequential design with quantitative data collected in the initial phase, followed by qualitative data
Exploratory sequential designs	Used when qualitative results need to be tested or generalized or for theory development or instrument development	Sequential design with qualitative data collected in the initial phase, followed by quantitative data
Multiphasic	Useful in comprehensive program evaluations by addressing a set of incremental research questions focused on a central objective	Combines the concurrent and/ or sequential collection of quantitative and qualitative data sets over multiple phases of a study

Though quantitative and qualitative studies both use systematic processes, they have distinct differences in their worldviews:

- Quantitative studies are objective; they test theory (deductive), involve the use of numbers, and produce findings that are meant to be generalizable.

- Qualitative studies are subjective; they generate knowledge through the process of induction, involve the use of words, and produce findings that are not meant to be generalizable.

After the EBP team has determined the level of research evidence based on study design, team members need to assess the quality of the evidence. To best assess quality, the team needs to understand how to interpret research evidence.

Interpreting Primary Research Evidence

To consider statistical information presented in reports of research evidence effectively, EBP team members need a basic understanding of a study's *validity, reliability,* and *precision*. Validity and reliability are the cornerstones of the scientific method. *Validity* refers to the credibility of the research—the extent to which the research measures what it claims to measure. *Reliability* refers to the consistency or repeatability of measurement. For example, a patient scale is off by 5 pounds. When the patient is weighed three times, the scale reads 137 every time (reliability). However, the weight is not the patient's true weight, because the scale isn't recording correctly (validity). Precision has to do with how to interpret statistical measures of central tendency (mean, median, and mode) and clinical and statistical significance (p-value, confidence interval).

Measures of Validity

The validity of research is important because if the study does not measure what is intended, the results won't effectively answer the aim of the research. There are two aspects of validity: internal and external. *Internal validity* is the degree to which observed changes in the dependent variable are caused by the experimental treatment or intervention rather than from other possible causes. An EBP team should question whether there are competing explanations for the observed results. Many factors pose threats to internal validity, all of which represent possible sources of bias. These include *investigator bias,* where a researcher subconsciously influences the study participants' responses. Another well-recognized threat to internal validity is the *Hawthorne effect,* in which participants alter their behavior because they are aware that they are being observed. Two other biases are *attrition bias* and *selection bias. Attrition bias* refers to the loss of subjects during a study and affects the representative nature of the sample. *Selection bias* exists in all nonrandomly selected samples.

External Validity

External validity refers to the likelihood that conclusions about research findings can be generalized to other settings or samples. External validity is a major concern with EBP when translating research into a real-world, clinical setting. An EBP team should question the degree to which study conclusions may reasonably hold true for its particular patient population and setting. Do the investigators state the participation rates of subjects and settings? Do they explain the intended target audience for the intervention or treatment? How representative is the sample of the population of interest?

Two strategies can improve the external validity of a research study: Ensure the representativeness of the study participants, and replicate the study in multiple sites that differ in dimensions such as size, setting, and staff skill set. If results are similar across these sites, this strengthens the external validity. The American Nurses Credentialing Center (ANCC) sponsors multisite studies in Magnet hospitals to foster participation in rigorous, large-scale research studies that contribute to nursing science. Information about the studies can be found at http://www.nursecredentialing.org/MagnetMultisiteStudyFAQ#researchteam-agreement.

Experimental studies are often high in internal validity because they are structured and control for extraneous variables. However, because of this, the generalizability of the results (external validity) may be limited. In contrast, nonexperimental and observational studies may be high in generalizability because the studies are conducted in real-world settings, but they are low on internal validity because of inability to control variables that may affect the results.

Measures of internal validity include *content validity, construct validity,* and *cross cultural validity*.

Content Validity

Content validity is the extent to which an instrument's content adequately measures a construct—whether an instrument has an appropriate sample of items for the construct being measured (Polit & Beck, 2017). An instrument's content validity is based on judgment. A panel of experts is often used to evaluate the content validity of a new instrument. Three issues are considered when experts are evaluating content validity. An assessment of the *relevance* of an item is the first issue. Experts are asked to rate an item on a 4-point scale of relevance to the content being measured or to a target population. The second consideration is the *comprehensiveness* of the items—that is, whether there are notable omissions to measuring the construct. The last issue to consider is *balance*—for example, in a multi-item scale, whether there are enough items to measure the construct to ensure internal consistency in the subscales (Polit & Beck, 2017).

Construct Validity

A *construct* is a way of defining something that can't be directly observed. Thus, *construct validity* is particularly important for an abstract construct such as motivation or intelligence. It concerns the measurement of abstract variables to ensure the correctness of assuming that what the investigators are measuring actually measures the construct of interest. If a researcher has taken careful steps noted in establishing content validity of the instrument, the construct validity will be strengthened (Polit & Beck, 2017). EBP teams often encounter discussion of construct validity when instruments are used in research studies. This refers to the degree to which the instrument measures the construct (or concept) under investigation. Questions a nurse may pose to get at threats to construct validity include these: "Did the researcher do a good job of defining the constructs? When the researchers say that they are measuring what they call fatigue, is that what they are really measuring?"

Cross-cultural validity is a type of construct validity. Cross-cultural validity is concerned with the degree to which the items of a translated or culturally adapted tool perform adequately and equivalently to the original instrument. Translation and adaption require high levels of statistical applications (Polit & Beck, 2017).

Measures of Reliability

The concept of *reliability* is used to describe the consistency of a set of measurements or of an instrument used to measure a construct. The question that is asked is, "Can the results be replicated if the test is repeated?" Reliability refers, in essence, to the repeatability of a test. For example, variation in measurements may exist when nurses use patient care equipment such as blood pressure cuffs or glucometers. Two methods used to measure reliability include test-retest reliability and interrater reliability. Test-retest reliability is done by administrating a measure to the same people on two occasions. If the difference in a person's scores is small, reliability is high. A second method to test reliability is interrater reliability, which involves having two or more observers independently apply an instrument to the same people.

Measures of Precision

Precision language describes populations and characteristics of populations. An EBP team should be quite familiar with measures of *central tendency* (mean, median, and mode) and *variation* (standard deviation). The *mean* denotes the average value and is used with numerical data. Although a good measure of central tendency in normal distributions, the mean is misleading in cases involving skewed (asymmetric) distributions and extreme scores. The *median,* the number that lies at the midpoint of a distribution of values, is less sensitive to extreme scores and is, therefore, of greater use in skewed distributions. The *mode* is the most frequently occurring value and is the only measure of central tendency used with categorical data. *Standard deviation* is a measure of variability that denotes the spread of the distribution and indicates the average variation of values from the mean.

Another measure of precision is *statistical significance,* which indicates whether findings are due to chance. The classic measure of statistical significance, the *p-value,* is a probability range from 0 to 1. The smaller the p-value (the closer it is to 0), the more likely the result is statistically significant and reflects an actual association or difference between variables/groups. The p-value is influenced by two factors: the sample size and the magnitude of the difference between groups (effect size) (Sullivan & Feinn, 2012). For example, if the sample size is large enough (e.g., 8,000), the results will almost always show a significant p-value, even if the effect size is small or clinically insignificant. In these instances, it may not be justifiable or time efficient to translate these results into practice. In nursing literature, the p-value for determining statistical significance is generally set at $p < 0.05$. Though p-values indicate statistical significance (i.e., the results are not due to chance), effect sizes increase readers' comprehension of the size of the differences found (clinical significance). Nursing research results are increasingly reporting *effect sizes* (clinical significance) and *confidence intervals* (precision measure for effect size) to more fully interpret results and guide decisions for translation.

Effect size is an important concept in EBP because it provides a common metric for summarizing evidence in meta-analysis. When combining studies in a meta-analysis, the effect size measures the strength of the relationship or association between variables in the research studies' combined populations. In quantitative studies other than meta-analysis, effect size is a more precise measure of the magnitude of the difference between groups (Sullivan & Feinn, 2012). Both are essential to the interpretation of results. An effect may be the result of a treatment, a decision, an intervention, or a program. The most commonly used estimate of the size of an intervention effect is *Cohen's d*, whereby 0.8 is considered to be a large effect, 0.5 is interpreted as a medium effect, and 0.2 equates to a small effect (Cohen, 1988). Consider that an experimental group of 20 new graduates is given a competency test on assessment of cardiac function after having a simulation experience. Their average score is 80 with a standard deviation (SD) of 10; the control group, which did not have a simulation experience, scores 75 with a standard deviation of 12. In this example of two independent groups, the effect size is calculated as follows ([*d = mean 1–mean 2/ SD of either group*]): 80 minus 75 divided by 10 equals 0.5, which is a medium effect size.

Confidence intervals (CI) address one key EBP question for appraising the evidence: How precise is the estimate of effects (Polit, 2010)? What exactly is the *confidence interval* (CI)? This measure of precision is an estimate of a range of values within which the actual value lies. The CI contains an upper limit and a lower limit. A 95% CI is the range of values within which an investigator can be 95% confident that the actual values in a given population fall within the upper and lower limits of the range of values. Consider a study on the effect of sucrose analgesia used to manage pain during venipuncture in newborn screening

(Taddio, Shah, & Katz, 2009). The researchers found that sucrose-treated infants had significantly lower pain scores during post-venipuncture diaper change than did water-treated infants (mean difference: −1.4 (95% CI: −2.4 to −0.4)). With repeated measurement of the population, the researchers would expect to find (with a 95% degree of certainty) consistent differences in neonatal pain scores, with the mean falling between −2.4 and −0.4. If the confidence interval includes 0, there is no difference or association between the variables/groups.

Appraising the Level and Quality of Research Evidence

The use of rating scales assists the critical appraisal of evidence. Rating scales present a structured way to differentiate evidence of varying levels and quality. The underlying assumption is that recommendations from higher levels of evidence of high quality would be more likely to represent best practices. Table 6.7 presents the rating hierarchy used in the Johns Hopkins Nursing Evidence-Based Practice (JHNEBP) process to evaluate the level of research evidence. Table 6.8 presents the JHNEBP rating guide for quantitative research evidence. (See also Appendix D for quality ratings for qualitative and mixed methods research evidence.)

Table 6.7   Rating Hierarchy for Level of Research Evidence

LEVEL	TYPE OF EVIDENCE
I	An experimental study, randomized controlled trial (RCT), explanatory mixed methods with only level I quantitative study, or systematic review of RCTs, with or without meta-analysis
II	A quasi-experimental study, explanatory mixed methods with only level II quantitative study, or systematic review of a combination of RCTs and quasi-experimental studies, or quasi-experimental studies only, with or without meta-analysis
III	A quantitative nonexperimental study; explanatory mixed methods with only level III quantitative study; exploratory, convergent, or multiphasic mixed methods studies; systematic review of a combination of RCTs, quasi-experimental, and nonexperimental studies, or nonexperimental studies only; or qualitative study or systematic review of qualitative studies, with or without a meta-synthesis

Table 6.8   Quality Rating for Quantitative Research Evidence

Grade	Research Evidence
A: High	Consistent, generalizable results; sufficient sample size for study design; adequate control; definitive conclusions; consistent recommendations based on comprehensive literature review that includes thorough reference to scientific evidence
B: Good	Reasonably consistent results; sufficient sample size for the study design; some control; fairly definitive conclusions; reasonably consistent recommendations based on fairly comprehensive literature review that includes some reference to scientific evidence
C: Low or Major flaw	Little evidence with inconsistent results; insufficient sample size for the study design; conclusions cannot be drawn

Grading the Quality of Research Evidence

The large numbers of checklists and rating instruments available for grading the quality of research studies presents a challenge to an EBP team. Tools to appraise the quality of scientific evidence usually contain explicit criteria with varying degrees of specificity according to the evidence type. EBP teams often do not have the comprehensive knowledge of methodological strengths and limitations required to interpret these criteria. An EBP team needs to involve someone with knowledge of interpretation of research and statistics—often a nurse with a doctoral degree—to guide them through the process.

Because the development of any EBP skill set is evolutionary, the JHNEBP model uses a broadly defined quality rating scale. This provides structure for the EBP team yet allows for the application of critical-thinking skills specific to the team's knowledge and experience. The application of this scale, shown in Table 6.8, accommodates qualitative judgments related to both research and nonresearch evidence.

Judgments of quality should be relative. At any given point in the process, each individual or group applies the same interpretation to the body of evidence.

As the group gains experience in reading and appraising research, the members' comfort level in making this determination will likely improve.

Meta-Analyses (Level I Evidence)

The strength of the evidence on which recommendations are made within a meta-analytic study depends on the design and quality of studies included in the meta-analysis as well as the design of the meta-analysis itself. Factors to consider include sampling criteria of the primary studies included in the analysis, quality of the primary studies, and variation in study outcomes between studies.

First, the EBP team looks at the types of research designs (level of evidence) included in the meta-analysis. Meta-analyses containing only randomized controlled trials are Level I evidence. Some meta-analyses include data from quasi-experimental or nonexperimental studies; hence, evidence would be at a level commensurate with the lowest level of research design included (e.g., if the meta-analysis included experimental and quasi-experimental studies, the meta-analysis would be Level II).

Second, the team should look at the quality of the individual studies included in the meta-analysis. For an EBP team to evaluate evidence obtained from a meta-analysis, the report of the meta-analysis must be detailed enough for the reader to understand the studies included.

Third, the team should assess the quality of the meta-analysis. The discussion section should include an overall summary of the findings, the magnitude of the effect, the number of studies, and the combined sample size. The discussion should present the overall quality of the evidence and consistency of findings (Polit & Beck, 2017). The discussion should include a recommendation for future research to improve the evidence base.

Experimental Studies (Level I Evidence)

Level I evidence, the highest in the rating hierarchy, is derived from a well-designed RCT on the question of interest (refer to Table 6.7). Level I evidence is also derived from a meta-analysis of RCTs that support the same findings in different samples of the same population. Internal validity, discussed earlier in this chapter, refers to the extent to which inferences regarding cause and effect are true. True experiments have a high degree of internal validity because manipulation and random assignment enables researchers to rule out most alternative explanations of results (Polit & Beck, 2017). In experimental designs, researchers still need to consider contamination between treatments. Subject mortality may affect the study. There may also be different dropout rates between experimental and control groups. This may be a threat particularly if the experimental treatment was painful or time-consuming. Participants remaining in the study may differ from those who dropped out. Even with strong research designs, it is important to assess the nature of possible biases. Selection biases should be assessed by comparing groups on pretest data (Polit & Beck, 2017). If there are no pretest measures, groups should be compared on demographic and disease variables such as age, health status, and ethnicity. If there are multiple points of data collection, attrition biases are important to assess by comparing those who did or did not complete the intervention. EBP groups want to analyze carefully how the researcher addresses possible sources of bias.

External validity refers to the extent that results will hold true across different subjects, settings, and procedures. The most frequent criticism by clinicians of RCTs is lack of external validity. Results from an RCT that has internal validity may be clinically limited if it lacks external validity—that is, if results cannot be applied to the relevant population. Questions a team may pose to uncover potential threats to external validity include, "How confident are we that the study findings can transfer from the sample to the entire population? Are the study conditions as close as possible to real-world situations? Did subjects have inherent differences even before manipulation of the independent variable (selection bias)? Are participants responding in a certain way because they know they are being observed (the Hawthorne effect)? Are there researcher behaviors or characteristics that may influence the subject's responses (experimenter effect)? In multi-institutional studies, are there variations in how study coordinators at various sites managed the trial?

Quasi-Experimental Studies (Level II Evidence)

The evidence gained from well-designed, quasi-experimental studies is lower than that of experimental studies. Quasi-experimental studies are indicated when ethical considerations, practical issues, and feasibility prohibit the conduct of RCTs. For that reason, the evidence rating for a well-designed quasi-experimental study is Level II (refer to Table 6.7).

As with experimental studies, threats to internal validity for quasi-experimental studies include maturation, testing, and instrumentation, with the additional threats of history and selection (Polit & Beck, 2017). The occurrence of external events during the study (threat of history) can affect a subject's response to the investigational intervention or treatment. Additionally, when groups are not assigned randomly, preexisting differences between the groups can affect the outcome. Questions the EBP team may pose to uncover potential threats to internal validity include, "Did some event occur during the course of the study that may have influenced the results of the study? Are there processes occurring within subjects over the course of the study because of the passage of time (maturation) rather than as a result of the experimental intervention? Could the pretest have influenced the subject's performance on the posttest? Were the measurement instruments and procedures the same for both points of data collection?"

In terms of external validity, threats associated with sampling design, such as patient selection and characteristics of nonrandomized patients, affect the general findings. External validity improves if the researcher uses random selection of subjects, even if random assignment to groups is not possible.

Nonexperimental and Qualitative Studies (Level III Evidence)

The evidence gained from well-designed, nonexperimental and qualitative studies is the lowest in the research hierarchy (Level III). Questions of internal validity do not apply when reviewing descriptive designs (quantitative or qualitative).

When looking for potential threats to external validity in quantitative nonexperimental studies, the EBP team can pose the questions described under experimental and quasi-experimental studies. In addition, the team may ask further questions such as, "Did the researcher attempt to control for extraneous variables with the use of careful subject-selection criteria? Did the researcher attempt to minimize the potential for socially acceptable responses by the subject? Did the study rely on documentation as the source of data? In methodological studies (developing, testing, and evaluating research instruments and methods), were the test subjects selected from the population for which the test will be used? Was the survey response rate high enough to generalize findings to the target population? For historical research studies, are the data authentic and genuine?"

Qualitative studies offer many challenges with respect to the question of validity. A number of ways to determine validity, or rigor, in qualitative research have been postulated. Four common approaches to establish rigor (Saumure & Given, 2012) are:

- *Transparency,* or how clear the research process has been explained
- *Credibility*, or the extent to which data are representative
- *Dependability*, or that other researchers would draw the same or similar conclusions when looking at the data
- *Reflexivity*, or how the researcher has reported the ways in which they were involved in the research and may have influenced the study results

Issues of rigor in qualitative research are complex, so the EBP team should appraise how well the researchers discuss how they determined validity for the particular study.

Meta-Syntheses (Level III Evidence)

Evaluating and synthesizing qualitative research presents many challenges. It is not surprising that EBP teams may feel at a loss in assessing the quality of meta-synthesis. Approaching these reviews from a broad perspective enables the team to look for indicators of quality that both quantitative and qualitative summative research techniques have in common.

Explicit search strategies, inclusion and exclusion criteria, methodological details (of not only the included studies but also the conduct of the meta-synthesis itself), and reviewer management of study quality should all be noted. Similar to other summative modalities, a "meta-synthesis should be undertaken by a team of experts since the application of multiple perspectives to the processes of study appraisal, coding, charting, mapping, and interpretation may result in additional insights, and thus in a more complete interpretation of the subject of the review" (Jones, 2004, p. 277).

EBP teams need to keep in mind that judgments related to study strengths and weaknesses as well as to the suitability of recommendations for the target population are both context-specific and dependent on the question asked. Some conditions or circumstances, such as clinical setting or time of day, are relevant to determining the applicability of a particular recommended intervention.

Rating Strength of Research Evidence

Research evidence, when well executed (of good to high quality), is generally given a higher strength rating than other types of evidence. When appraising individual research studies, two major components come into play: study design (level) and study quality (methods and execution), with particular attention given to study limitations. When synthesizing overall evidence, important criteria are quality, consistency of evidence, and applicability to population or setting of interest.

Tips for Reading Research

Teams engaging in EBP activities should be educated readers and interpreters of research publications. The completeness of a research report and the reader's ability to understand the meaning of terms used in the report can help or hinder an EBP team's efforts. Though standards exist for writing research articles, the degree to which journals demand adherence to these standards varies. Classic elements of published research include the *title, abstract, introduction, method, results, discussion,* and *conclusion* (Lunsford & Lunsford, 1996). Another organization format is IMRAD, which organizes material into four sections:

introduction, method, results, and discussion. Readers will find that research reports do not always clearly delineate these sections with headers, although the elements may still be present. For example, typically, the introduction or conclusion of a research report has no heading. Additionally, nurses need to develop a strategy for reading research articles with a critical eye. A sequential strategy is to read the title, then the abstract, then jump to the conclusion, and then decide whether you want to read the article. If so, then go back to the beginning and read the article in its entirety.

The Title

When searching for written research evidence, an EBP team encounters a listing of potential titles. The title presents a starting point in determining whether the article has the potential to be included in an EBP review. Ideally, the title should be informative and help the reader understand what type of study is being reported. A well-chosen title states what was done, to whom it was done, and how it was done. Consider the title "Effects of a peer-assisted tai-chi-qigong programme on social isolation and psychological wellbeing in Chinese hidden elders: a pilot randomized controlled trial" (Chan, Yu, Choi, Chan, & Wong, 2016). The reader is immediately apprised of what was done (peer-assisted programme intervention), to whom it was done (Chinese hidden elders), and how it was done (a randomized controlled trial).

Often, articles germane to an EBP question are skipped because the title does not give a clue to its relevance. For example, consider the title "Urinary Tract Infection Rates Associated with Re-Use of Catheters in Clean Intermittent Catheterization of Male Veterans" (Kannankeril, Lam, Reyes, & McCartney, 2011). Although the reader can get the idea that the article concerns urinary tract infection rates in male veterans who undergo clean intermittent catheterization (*what* and *in whom*), the title gives no indication that this is a report of a nonexperimental research study using a descriptive design. The title is more reflective of an opinion piece than a research report.

The Abstract

The abstract is usually located after the title and author section and is graphically set apart by use of a box, shading, or italics. The abstract is a brief description of the problem, methods, and findings of the study (Polit & Beck, 2017). The abstract provides the information needed to quickly screen the relevance of the study to the EBP topic.

The Introduction

If the abstract appears to be relevant, the team should move on to an examination of the introduction. The introduction contains the background as well as a problem statement that tells why the investigators have chosen to conduct the particular study. Background is best presented within the context of a current literature review, and the author should identify the knowledge gap between what is known and what the study seeks to find out (or answer). A clear, direct statement of purpose should be included as well as a statement of expected results or hypotheses. The statement of purpose is often, although not always, located immediately before the article's first main heading.

The Method

This section describes how a study is conducted (study procedures) in sufficient detail so that readers can replicate the study, if desired. For example, if the intervention was administration of a placebo, the nature of the placebo should be stated. An investigator should identify the intended study population and provide a description of inclusion and exclusion criteria. How subjects were recruited and demographic characteristics of those who actually took part in the study should be included. In addition, if instrumentation was used, the method section should present evidence of instrument quality even if well-known published tools are used. An acknowledgement of ethical review for research studies involving human subjects should also be presented. Finally, the report should contain a description of how data were collected and analyzed.

The Results

Study results list the findings of the data analysis and should not contain commentary. Give particular attention to figures and tables, which are the heart of most papers. Look to see whether results report statistical versus clinical significance, and look up unfamiliar terminology, symbols, or logic.

The Discussion

Results should be tied to material in the introduction. The research findings should be discussed and meaning given to the results. The main weaknesses or limitations of the study should be identified with the actions taken to minimize them, and the broad implications of the findings should be stated.

The reviewer should be cautioned that writers may use language to sway the reader. In his classic discussion on reading research, Graham (1957) notes that researchers can overstate their findings or use an assertive sentence in a way that makes their statement of findings sound like a well-established fact. (Critically view vague expressions similar to "It is generally believed that...")

The Conclusion

The conclusion should contain a brief restatement of the experimental results and implications of the study (Lunsford & Lunsford, 1996). If the conclusion is not called out by a separate header, it usually falls at the end of the discussion section.

The Overall Report

The parts of the research article should be highly interconnected and provide sufficient information so that the reviewer can make an informed judgment about the connections. Any hypotheses should flow directly from the review of literature. Results should support arguments presented in the discussion and conclusion sections.

An EBP team should be aware of duplicate publications—that is, more than one publication that reports findings from the same research study. "Duplicate publication of original research is particularly problematic, since it can result in inadvertent double counting or inappropriate weighting of the results of a single study, which distorts the available evidence" (International Committee of Medical Journal Editors, 2010, IIID2).

A Practical Tool for Appraising Research Evidence

The Research Evidence Appraisal Tool (see Appendix E) gauges the level and quality of research evidence. The tool contains questions to guide the team in determining the level of evidence and the quality of the primary studies included in the review. Strength (level and quality) is higher (Level I) with evidence from at least one well-designed (quality), randomized controlled trial (RCT) than from at least one well-designed quasi-experimental (Level II), nonexperimental (Level III), or qualitative (Level III) study. The tool also contains questions to guide appraisal and to determine the quality of the research.

An EBP team can use the Individual Evidence Summary Tool (see Appendix G) to summarize key findings from each of the individual pieces of evidence that answers the EBP question. This enables team members to view pertinent information related to each source (author, evidence type, sample, setting, findings that answer the EBP question, limitations, level of evidence, and quality ratings) in one document.

An EBP team can use the Synthesis and Recommendations Tool (see Appendix H) to document the quantity or number of evidence sources for each level of evidence, determine the overall quality rating for each level, and synthesize findings to conclude if practice, process, or system changes should be made. The team's final recommendations are listed at the bottom of the tool. A guide to how to synthesize evidence is provided in Appendix H.

Recommendation for Nurse Leaders

Knowledge gained from research studies is valuable only to the extent that it is shared with others and appropriately translated into practice. Professional standards have long held that nurses need to integrate the best available evidence, including research findings, into practice decisions. Research articles can be intimidating to novice and expert nurses alike. Because many EBP teams do not have the skill set to fully judge the proper use of statistics in the studies under review, it is highly recommended that teams draw on research texts, mentors, or experts to guide the process.

Nurse leaders can best support EBP by providing clinicians with the knowledge and skills necessary to appraise research evidence. Only through continuous learning can clinicians gain the confidence needed to incorporate evidence gleaned from research into the day-to-day care of individual patients.

Summary

This chapter arms EBP teams with practical information to guide the appraisal of research evidence, a task that is often difficult for nonresearchers. An overview of the various types of research evidence is presented, including attention to individual research studies and summaries of multiple research studies. Tips for reading research reports are provided, along with guidance on how to appraise the level and quality of research evidence.

References

Agency for Healthcare Research and Quality (AHRQ). (2011). Evidence-based Practice Centers. Retrieved from http://www.ahrq.gov/clinic/epc

Al-Yateem, N. (2013). Guidelines for the transition from child to adult cystic fibrosis care. *Nursing Children and Young People, 25*(5), 29–34.

Back, J., Jin, Y., Jin, T., & Lee, S. (2016). Development and validation of an automated sepsis risk assessment system. *Journal of Nursing & Health, 39,* 317–327.

Beck, C. T., & Harrison, L. (2016). Mixed-methods research in the discipline of nursing. *Advances in Nursing Science, 39*(3), 224–234.

Belli, G. (2009). Analysis and interpretation of nonexperimental studies. In Lapan, S. D., & Quartaroli, M. T. (Eds.). *Research Essentials: An Introduction to Designs and Practices,* pp. 59–77. Retrieved from http://media.wiley.com/product_data/excer pt/95/04701810/0470181095-1.pdf

Birks, M., & Mills, J. (2015). *Grounded theory: A practical guide* (2nd ed.).: Thousand Oaks, CA: SAGE.

Bourgault, A., Heath, J., Hooper, V., Sole, M., Waller, J., & NeSmith, E. (2014). Factors influencing critical-care nurses' adoption of the AACN practice alert on verification of feeding tube placement. *American Journal of Critical Care, 23*(2), 134–144.

Centre for Evidence-Based Intervention (CEBI). (n.d.). Retrieved from https://www.cebi.ox.ac.uk/for-practitioners/what-is-good-evidence/how-to-read-a-forest-plot.html

Chan, A., Yu, D., Choi, K., Chan, H., & Wong, E. (2016). Effects of a peer-assisted tai-chi-qigong programme on social isolation and psychological wellbeing in Chinese hidden elders: A pilot randomized controlled trial. *The Lancet, 388*(S23).

Chunfeng Wang, C., & Geale, S. K. (2015). The power of story: Narrative inquiry as a methodology in nursing research. *International Journal of Nursing Sciences, 2*(2), 195–198.

The Cochrane Collaboration. (2016). The Cochrane Collaboration. Retrieved from http://www.cochrane.org

Cohen, J. (1988). *Statistical power analysis for the behavioral sciences.* New York: Academic Press.

Creswell, J. W. (2014). *A concise introduction to mixed methods research.* Thousand Oaks, CA: SAGE.

Curtis, P., & Northcott, A. (2017). The impact of single and shared rooms on family-centered care in children's hospitals. *Journal of Clinical Nursing, 26*(11–12), 1584–1596.

Dabney, B., & Kalisch, B. (2015). Nurse staffing levels and patient-reported missed nursing care. *Journal of Nursing Care Quality, 30*(4), 306–312.

de Chesnay, M. (2014). *Nursing research using ethnography: Qualitative designs and methods in nursing.* New York: Springer Publishing Company.

Dybitz, S. B., Thompson, S., Molotsky, S., & Stuart, B. (2011). Prevalence of diabetes and the burden of comorbid conditions among elderly nursing home patients. *American Journal of Geriatric Pharmacotherapy, 9*(4), 212–223.

EPC Evidence-Based Reports. Content last reviewed August 2016. Agency for Healthcare Research and Quality, Rockville, MD. Retrieved from http://www.ahrq.gov/research/findings/evidence-based-reports/index.html

Fildes, A., Charlton, J., Rudisill, C., Littlejohns, P., Prevost, T., & Gulliford, M. (2015). Probability of an obese person attaining normal body weight: Cohort study using electronic health records. *American Journal of Public Health, 105,* e54–e59.

Flores, D., Leblanc, N., & Barroso, J. (2016). Enrolling and retaining human immunodeficiency virus (HIV) patients in their care: A metasynthesis of qualitative studies. *International Journal of Nursing Studies, 62,* 126–136.

Gordis, L. (2009). *Epidemiology.* Philadelphia, PA: Saunders Elsevier.

Graham, C. D. (1957). *A dictionary of useful research phrases.* Originally published in *Metal Progress, 71*(5). Retrieved from http://www.ece.vt.edu/thou/Dictionary%20of%20Useful%20Research%20Phrases.htm

Higgins, J. P. T., & Green, S. (Eds.). (2015). *Cochrane Handbook for Systematic Reviews of Interventions* Version 5.3.0 (updated October 2015). The Cochrane Collaboration. Available from http://methods.cochrane.org/qi/supplemental-handbook-guidance

Hyatt, K. S., Davis, L. L., & Barroso, J. (2015). Finding the new normal: Accepting changes after combat-related mild traumatic brain injury. *Journal of Nursing Scholarship. 47*(4), 300–309.

Institute of Medicine. (2011). *Finding what works in health care standards for systematic reviews.* Washington, D.C.: National Academy of Sciences.

International Committee of Medical Journal Editors. (2010). Uniform requirements for manuscripts submitted to biomedical journals: Writing and editing for biomedical publications. Retrieved from http://www.ICMJE.org

Jones, M. L. (2004). Application of systematic review methods to qualitative research: Practical issues. *Journal of Advanced Nursing, 48*(3), 271–278.

Kannankeril, A. J., Lam, H. T., Reyes, E. B., & McCartney, J. (2011). Urinary tract infection rates associated with re-use of catheters in clean intermittent catheterization of male veterans. *Urologic Nursing, 31*(1), 41–48.

Kiecolt-Glaser, J., Bennett, J., Amdrodge, R., Peng, J., Shapiro, C., Malarkey, W.,…Glaser, R. (2014). Yoga's impact on inflammation, mood, and fatigue in breast cancer survivors: A randomized controlled trial. *Journal of Clinical Oncology, 32*(10), 1040–1049.

Labrague, L., & McEnroe-Petitte, D. (2014). Influence of music on preoperative anxiety and physiologic parameters in women undergoing gynecologic surgery. *Clinical Nursing Research,* 1–17.

LaFond, C. M., Van Hulle Vincent, C., Oosterhouse, K., & Wilkie, D. J. (2016). Nurses' beliefs regarding pain in critically ill children: A mixed-methods study. *Journal of Pediatric Nursing. 31*(6), 691–700.

Lu, C. Y. (2009). Observational studies: A review of study designs, challenges, and strategies to reduce confounding. *The International Journal of Clinical Practice, 63*(5), 691–697.

Lunsford, T. R., & Lunsford, B. R. (1996). Research forum: How to critically read a journal research article. *Journal of Prosthetics and Orthotics, 8*(1), 24–31.

MacWilliams, K., Hughes, J., Aston, M., Field, S., & Wight Moffatt, F. (2016). Understanding the experience of miscarriage in the emergency department. *Journal of Emergency Nursing.* [Epub ahead of print].

Mazanec, S. R., Daly, B. J., Douglas, S., & Musil, C. (2011). Predictors of psychosocial adjustment during the post-radiation treatment transition. *Western Journal of Nursing Research, 33*(4), 540–559.

McConnell, B., & Moroney T. (2015). Involving relatives in ICU patient care: Critical nurse challenges. *Journal of Clinical Nursing. 24*(7–8), 991–998.

Melnyk, B. and Newhouse R. (2014) Evidence-based practice versus evidence-informed practice: A debate that could stall forward momentum in improving healthcare quality, safety, patient outcomes and cost. *Worldviews on Evidence-Based Nursing. 11*(6), 347–349.

Mills, J., Chamberlain-Salaun, J., Harrison, H., Yates, K., & O'Shea, A. (2016). Retaining early career registered nurses: a case study. *BMC Nursing,* 15, 57.

Nam S., Janson, S., Stotts, N., Chesla, C., & Kroon, L. (2012). Effect of culturally tailored diabetes education in ethnic minorities with type 2 diabetes a meta-analysis. *Journal of Cardiovascular Nursing, 27*(6), 505–518.

Noblit, G. W., & Hare, R. D. (1988). *Meta-ethnography: Synthesizing qualitative studies*. Newbury Park, CA: SAGE.

Polit, D. F. (2010). *Statistics and data analysis for nursing research*. (2nd ed.). Upper Saddle River, NJ: Pearson Education.

Polit, D. F., & Beck, C. T. (2017). *Nursing research: Generating and assessing evidence for nursing practice* (10th ed.). Philadelphia: Lippincott Williams & Wilkens.

Reed, R., Rowe, J. & Barnes, M. (2015). Midwifery practice during birth: Ritual companionship. *Women and Birth*. 29, 269–278.

Roberts, C. A. (2010). Unaccompanied hospitalized children: A review of the literature and incidence study. *Journal of Pediatric Nursing*, 25(6), 470–476.

Roberts, D., & Dalziel S. R. (2006). Antenatal corticosteroids for accelerating fetal lung maturation for women at risk of preterm birth. *Cochrane Database of Systematic Reviews*, (3). Art. No.: CD004454.

Sandelowski, M. (2000). Whatever happened to qualitative description? *Research in Nursing & Health*, 23(4), pp. 334–340.

Sangster-Gormley, E., Griffith, J., Schreiber, R., & Borycki, E. (2015). Using a mixed-methods design to examine nurse practitioner integration in British Columbia. *Nurse Researcher*, 22(6), 16–21.

Saumure, K., & Given, L. M. (2012). Rigor in qualitative research. In Given, L. M. (Ed.) *The SAGE Encyclopedia of Qualitative Research Methods*. Thousand Oaks, CA: SAGE.

Saunders, H., & Vehviläinen-Julkunen, K. (2016). Evidence-based practice and job-related nurse outcomes at Magnet-aspiring, Magnet-conforming, and non-Magnet university hospitals in Finland: A comparison study. *Journal of Nursing Administration*, 46(10), 513–520.

Shafir, A., Garrigues, S. K., Schenker, Y., Leff, B., Neil, J., & Ritchie, C. (2016). Homebound patient and caregiver perceptions of quality of care in home-based primary care: A qualitative study. *Journal of the American Geriatrics Society*. 64(8), 1622–1627.

Stake, R. (1995). *The art of case study research*. Thousand Oaks, CA: SAGE.

Stickney, C., Ziniel, S., Brett, M., & Truog, R. (2014). Family participation during intensive care unit rounds: Attitudes and experiences of parents and healthcare providers in a tertiary pediatric intensive care unit. *American Journal of Pediatrics*, 164, 402–406.

Sullivan, G. M., & Feinn, R. (2012). Using effect size—or why the p value is not enough. *Journal of Graduate Medical Education*, 4(3), 279–282.

Taddio, A., Shah, V., & Katz, J. (2009). Reduced infant response to a routine care procedure after sucrose analgesia. *Pediatrics*, 123(3), e425–429.

Worldviews on Evidence-Based Nursing. (2016). Retrieved from http://www.nursingsociety.org/learn-grow/publications/worldviews-on-evidence-based-nursing

Evidence Appraisal: Nonresearch

One distinguishing feature of evidence-based practice (EBP) is the inclusion of multiple sources of evidence. When research evidence does not exist or is insufficient to answer the practice question, nurses have a range of nonresearch evidence to draw from that has the potential to inform their practice.

Such evidence includes personal, aesthetic, and ethical ways of knowing (Carper, 1978)—for example, the expertise, experience, and values of individual practitioners, patients, and patients' families. For the purposes of this chapter, nonresearch evidence is divided into summaries of evidence (clinical practice guidelines, consensus or position statements, literature and integrative reviews); organizational experience (quality improvement and financial data); expert opinion (commentary or opinion, case reports); community standards; clinician experience; and consumer preferences. This chapter:

- Describes types of nonresearch evidence
- Explains strategies for evaluating such evidence

- Recommends approaches for building nurses' capacity to appraise non-research evidence to inform their practice

Summaries of Research Evidence

Summaries of research evidence such as clinical practice guidelines, consensus or position statements, integrative reviews, and literature reviews are excellent sources of evidence relevant to practice questions. These forms of evidence review and summarize all research, not just experimental studies. They are not classified as research evidence because summaries of research evidence are often not comprehensive and may not include an appraisal of study quality.

Clinical Practice Guidelines and Consensus/Position Statements (Level IV Evidence)

Clinical practice guidelines (CPGs) are systematically developed statements that guide clinical practice and evidence-based decision-making (Polit & Beck, 2017). CPGs, which are recommendations that synthesize available experimental and clinical evidence with bedside experience, are open to comment, criticism, and updating (Deresinski & File, 2011). Consensus or position statements (CSs) are similar to CPGs in that they are systematically developed recommendations that may or may not be supported by research. CSs are broad statements of best practice; are most often meant to guide members of a professional organization in decision-making; and do not provide specific algorithms for practice (Lopez-Olivio, Kallen, Ortiz, Skidmore, & Suarez-Almazor, 2008).

The past two decades have seen an exponential increase in CPGs and CSs. To help practitioners determine the quality of CPGs, the Institute of Medicine (IOM) identified eight desirable attributes, which include validity; reliability and reproducibility; clinical applicability; clinical flexibility; clarity; documentation; development by a multidisciplinary process; and plans for review (IOM, 1992). Many of these attributes were absent from published guidelines, resulting in the *Conference on Guideline Standardization* to promote guideline quality and to facilitate implementation (Shiffman et al., 2003). The *Appraisal of Guidelines Research and Evaluation (AGREE) Collaboration*, using a guideline appraisal instrument with documented reliability and validity, found that the availability of background information was the strongest predictor of guideline quality and that high-quality guidelines were more often produced by government-supported organizations or a structured, coordinated program (Fervers et al., 2005). The AGREE instrument, revised in 2013, now has 23 items and is organized into six domains (The AGREE Research Trust, 2013; Brouwers et al., 2010):

1. Scope and purpose

2. Stakeholder involvement

3. Rigor of development

4. Clarity of presentation

5. Applicability

6. Editorial independence

The National Guideline Clearinghouse (NGC), an initiative of the Agency for Healthcare Research and Quality (AHRQ), U.S. Department of Health and Human Services, is another excellent source of high-quality guidelines and is known for its rigorous standards. The NGC recently revised the criteria designed to ensure rigor in developing and maintaining published guidelines (NGC, 2013). The revised criteria stipulate that the guidelines:

- Contain systematically developed statements, including recommendations to optimize patient care and assist physicians and/or other healthcare practitioners and patients to make decisions

- Have been produced by a medical specialty association, relevant professional society, public or private organization, government agency, or healthcare organization or plan

- Be based on a systematic review of evidence

- Contain an assessment of the benefits and harms of recommended care and alternative care options

- Have the full text guideline available in English to the public upon request
- Be the most recent version published and have been developed, reviewed, or revised within the past five years

An example of a set of guidelines that meets the exacting requirements of the NGC is the "2013 ACC/AHA Guideline on the Treatment of Blood Cholesterol to Reduce Atherosclerotic Cardiovascular Risk in Adults: A Report of the American College of Cardiology/American Heart Association Task Force on Practice Guidelines" (Stone et al., 2014).

Despite these recommendations, guidelines still vary greatly in how they are developed and how the results are reported (Kuehn, 2011). In response to concern about the quality, two reports were released by the IOM to set standards for clinical practice guidelines (IOM, 2011). The IOM developed eight standard practices for creating CPGs (see Table 7.1). The IOM CPG standards describe the information that should be in the guidelines and development processes to be followed.

Table 7.1   Clinical Practice Guideline (CPG) Standards and Description

Standard	Description
Establish transparency.	Funding and development process should be publicly available.
Disclose conflict(s) of interest (COI).	Individuals who create guidelines and panel chairs should be free from conflicts of interest (COI). Funders are excluded from CPG development. All COIs of each Guideline Development Group member should be disclosed.
Balance membership of guideline development group.	Guideline developers should include multiple disciplines, patients, patient advocates, or patient consumer organizations.

Standard	Description
Use systematic reviews.	CPG developers should use systematic reviews that meet IOM's Standards for Systematic Reviews of Comparative Effectiveness Research.
Establish evidence foundations and rate strength of recommendations.	Rating has specified criteria for strength of recommendations.
Articulate recommendations.	Recommendations should follow a standard format and be worded so that compliance can be evaluated.
Include external reviewers.	External reviews should represent all relevant stakeholders, and their identity should be kept confidential. A draft of the CPG should be available to the public at the external review stage or directly afterward.
Update guidelines.	CPGs should be updated when new evidence suggests the need, and the CPG publication date, date of systematic evidence review, and proposed date for future review should be documented.

Literature Reviews (Level V Evidence)

Literature review is a broad term that generally refers to a summary of published literature without systematic appraisal of evidence quality or level. Traditional literature reviews are not confined to summaries of scientific literature; they can also present a narrative description of information from nonscientific literature, including reports of organizational experience and opinions of experts. Such reviews possess some of the desired attributes of a systematic review, but not the same standardized approach, appraisal, and critical review of the studies. For example, an author of a narrative review of research studies related to a particular question may describe comprehensive, even replicable, literature search strategies but neglect to appraise the quality of the studies discussed. Literature reviews also vary in completeness and often lack the intent of summarizing all available evidence on a topic (Grant & Booth, 2009).

An example of a narrative literature review is "The use and application of drama in nursing education—An integrative review of the literature" (Arveklev, Wigert, Berg, Burton, & Lepp, 2015), which draws information from published studies and reports effectiveness of drama in entry-level courses in nursing education.

Integrative Reviews (Level V Evidence)

Integrative reviews are the broadest form of summaries of research evidence. They summarize evidence that is a combination of research and theoretical literature and draw from manuscripts using varied methodologies (e.g., experimental, nonexperimental, qualitative). The purpose of an integrative review may vary widely and include summarizing evidence on a particular topic, reviewing theories, or defining concepts, among other topics. As with other summaries of evidence, well-defined and clearly presented search strategies are critical. Because diverse methodologies may be combined in an integrative review, quality evaluation or further analysis of data is complex. Unlike the literature review, however, an integrative review analyzes, compares themes, and notes gaps in the selected literature (Whittemore & Knafl, 2005).

An example of an integrative review is "An Integrative Review of Engaging Clinical Nurses in Nursing Research" (Scala, Price, & Day, 2016), which includes program evaluations, expert opinions, nonexperimental studies, and other papers using other methods to examine engaging clinical nurses in nursing research.

Interpreting Evidence from Summaries of Research Evidence

Despite efforts to ensure quality, the degree to which CPGs and CSs draw from existing evidence can fluctuate. Most guidelines are based on systematic reviews developed by experts whose charge is to arrive at specific clinical conclusions (IOM, 2001). Additionally, guidelines can lack the specificity needed to ensure consistent application across patients with the same clinical situation. Because the evidence base can be limited, or conflicting, the EBP team needs to exercise critical thinking and judgment when making recommendations.

Attention has also been paid to assessing equity in clinical practice guidelines. Equity concerns arise in groups potentially vulnerable to inequity because of residence, race, occupation, gender, religion, education, socioeconomic status, social network, and capital (Dans et al., 2007). When appropriate, an EBP team must consider the sociopolitical dimensions of applying CPGs to disadvantaged patient populations.

The age of the patient population is equally as important. Consider the anatomic, physiologic, and developmental differences between children and adults before applying published guidelines. Also, if possible, find a guideline specifically developed for children. For example, Black, Flynn, Smith, Thomas, and Wilkinson (2015) developed a pediatric airway-management guideline because only an adult guideline was available.

EBP teams also need to note that although groups of experts create these guidelines, which frequently carry a professional society's seal of approval, opinions that convert data to recommendations require subjective judgments that, in turn, leave room for error and bias (Mims, 2015). Potential conflicts of interest can be generated by financial interests, job descriptions, personal research interests, and previous experience. The IOM panel recommended that, whenever possible, individuals who create the guidelines should be free from conflicts of interest; if that is not possible, however, those individuals with conflicts of interest should make up a minority of the panel and should not serve as chairs or co-chairs (IOM, 2011).

Key elements to note when appraising Level IV evidence and rating evidence quality are identified in Table 7.2 and in the JHNEBP Nonresearch Evidence Appraisal Tool (see Appendix F).

Table 7.2   Desirable Attributes of Summative Documents Used to Answer an EBP Question

Attribute	Question
Applicability to phenomenon of interest	Does the summative document address the particular practice question of interest (same population, same setting)?
Comprehensiveness of search strategy	Do the authors identify search strategies that move beyond the typical databases, such as MEDLINE and CINAHL? Are published and unpublished works included?
Clarity of method	Do the authors clearly specify how decisions were made to include and exclude studies from the analysis and how data were analyzed?
Unity and consistency of findings	Is there cohesive organization of study findings so that meaningful separation and synthesis of relevant concepts are clear to the reader? Does the publication contain logically organized tables with consistent information relative to the applicability of findings?
Management of study quality	Do the authors clearly describe how the review addresses study quality?
Transparency of limitations	Are methodological limitations disclosed?
Believability of conclusions	Do the conclusions appear to be based on the evidence and capture the complexity of the clinical phenomenon?
Collective expertise	Were the review and synthesis done by a single individual with expertise or a group of experts?

Adapted from Whittemore (2005), Conn (2004), and Stetler et al. (1998).

Organizational Experience

Organizational experience often takes the form of quality improvement (QI) and financial or program evaluations. These sources of evidence can occur at any level in the organization and can be internal to an EBP team's organization or published reports from external organizations. Although they may be conducted within a framework of scientific inquiry and designed as research studies, most internal program evaluations are less rigorous (Level V). Frequently, they comprise pre- and/or post-implementation data at the organizational level accompanied by qualitative reports of personal satisfaction with the program. An example of a program evaluation is "Promoting Optimal Parenting and Children's Mental Health: A Preliminary Evaluation of the How-to Parenting Program" (Joussemet, Mageau, & Koestner, 2014), which evaluated the effectiveness of a parenting program in fostering optimal parenting and child mental health. This pre- and post-test method concluded that the How-to Parenting Program effectively improved parenting style and promoted children's mental health.

Quality Improvement Reports (Level V Evidence)

Quality improvement (QI) is a term that can be used interchangeably with quality management, performance improvement, total quality management, and continuous quality improvement (Yoder-Wise, 2014). These terms refer to ongoing efforts to improve the quality of care delivery and outcomes within an organization. QI is a cyclical method to examine workflows, processes, or systems within a specific organization. This information usually cannot be generalized beyond the organization. The organizational experience described here is distinctly different from quality-focused research or health services research intended to generalize results. Health services research uses experimental, quasi-experimental, non-experimental, and mixed-methods research designs (described in Chapter 6) and should be reviewed and appraised accordingly.

QI is a method of self-examination to inform improvement efforts at the local level. During their review of nonresearch evidence, EBP team members should examine internal QI data relating to the practice question as well as QI initiatives based on similar questions published by peer institutions. As organizations become more mature in their QI efforts, they become more rigorous in the approach, the analysis of results, and the use of established measures as metrics (Newhouse, Pettit, Poe, & Rocco, 2006). In contrast to research studies, the findings from QI studies are not meant to be generalized to other settings. Organizations that may benefit from the findings need to make decisions regarding implementation based on the characteristics of their organization.

QI reporting is an internal process; nevertheless, the desire to share the results from such projects is evident in the growing number of collaborative efforts targeting risk-prone issues. For example, the Institute of Healthcare Improvement (IHI) sponsored a learning and innovation network of quality-focused organizations working together to achieve improvement in healthcare areas such as perinatal care and the reduction of re-hospitalization. The IHI expanded these efforts and worked across organizational boundaries and engaged payers, state and national policymakers, patients, families, and caregivers at multiple care sites and clinical interfaces through the STate Action on Avoidable Rehospitalizations (STARR) Initiative (IHI, 2013). As the number of quality improvement reports has grown, so has concern about the quality of reporting. In an effort to reduce uncertainty about what information should be included in scholarly reports of health improvement, the Standards for Quality Improvement Reporting Excellence (SQUIRE: http://www.squire-statement.org) were published in 2008 and revised in 2015. The SQUIRE guidelines list and explain items that authors should consider including in a report of system-level work to improve healthcare (Ogrinc et al., 2015). Although evidence obtained from QI initiatives is not as strong as that obtained by scientific inquiry, the sharing of successful QI stories has the potential to identify future EBP questions, QI projects, and research studies external to the organization.

An example of a quality improvement project is a report from an emergency department (ED) and medical intensive care unit (MICU) on transfer time delays of critically ill patients from ED to MICU (Cohen et al., 2015). Using a clinical microsystems approach, the existing practice patterns were identified, and multiple causes that contributed to delays were determined. The Plan-Do-Study-Act model was applied in each intervention to reduce delays. The intervention reduced transfer time by 48% by improving coordination in multiple stages. This Level V evidence is from one institution that implemented a quality improvement project.

Financial Evaluation (Level V Evidence)

Financial and quality measures in healthcare facilities provide data to assess the cost associated with practice changes. Cost savings can be powerful information as the best practice is examined. An EBP team can find reports of cost effectiveness and economic evaluations (Level V) in published data or internal organizational reports. One example is "The Value of Reducing Hospital-Acquired Pressure Ulcer Prevalence." This study assessed the cost savings associated with implementing nursing approaches to prevent hospital-acquired pressure ulcers (HAPU) (Spetz, Brown, Aydin, Donaldson, 2013).

Terms used in the literature for projects dealing with finances include an *economic evaluation* that applies analytic techniques to identify, measure, and compare the costs and outcomes of two or more alternative programs or interventions (Centers for Disease Control and Prevention [CDC], 2007). A common economic evaluation of healthcare decision-making is a *cost-effectiveness analysis,* which compares costs of alternative interventions that produce a common health outcome. Although the results of such an analysis can provide justification for a program, empirical evidence can provide support for an increase in program funding or a switch from one program to another (CDC, 2007).

Financial data can be evaluated as listed on the JHNEBP Nonresearch Evidence Appraisal Tool. In reviewing a report, examine the aim, method, measures, results, and discussion for clarity. Carande-Kulis et al. (2000) recommend that standard inclusion criteria for economic studies have an analytic method and provide sufficient detail regarding the method and results. In assessing the quality of the economic study, the Community Guide "Economic Evaluation Abstraction Form" (2010) suggests that you ask the following questions:

- Was the study population well described?
- Was the question being analyzed well defined?
- Did the study define the time frame?

- Were data sources for all costs reported?

- Were data sources and costs appropriate with respect to the program and population being tested?

- Was the primary outcome measure clearly specified?

- Did outcomes include the effects or unintended outcomes of the program?

- Was the analytic model reported in an explicit manner?

- Were sensitivity analyses performed?

Not all studies that include cost analysis are strictly financial evaluations. When evaluating an article with a cost analysis, note that some articles may use rigorous designs and should be appraised using the Research Evidence Appraisal Tool (see Appendix E). An example of the use of a cost analysis is a report by Yang et al. (2015) that evaluates the impact of different nursing staffing models on patient safety, quality of care, and nursing costs. Results indicated that units with a 76% proportion of RNs made fewer medication errors and had a lower rate of ventilation weaning and that the units with a 92% RN proportion had a lower rate of bloodstream infections. The 76% and 92% RNs groups showed increased urinary tract infection and nursing costs (Yang, Hung, & Chen, 2015). After a review of this study, the EBP team would discover that this was actually a descriptive, retrospective cohort design study. Thus, it requires use of research appraisal criteria to judge the level and quality of evidence.

Expert Opinion (Level V Evidence)

The opinions of experts take the form of commentary articles, case reports, or letters to the editor. Expert opinion can also be written and in the form of a conversation with a recognized expert. External recognition (state, regional, national, international) that a professional is an expert is critical to determining the confidence an EBP team has in the expert's recommendations. Assessing expertise of an author of commentaries and opinion pieces requires another step. The EBP team can review the author's education, work, university affiliations, and publications on the topic; see whether others have cited the author's work; or see whether the author is a recognized speaker. For example, Netherwood, Skittrall, and Alexis (2014) provide an expert opinion on regulation of nursing assistants. This article could be rated high-quality because the authors are faculty members of a school of nursing and have additional publications on this topic. Their report is based on the literature with data supporting their opinion.

Case Report (Level V Evidence)

Case reports are commonly used in healthcare as a means of disseminating information on unusual clinical situations or scenarios, are used as educational tools, and are easily accessible. These reports present a summary or anecdotal description that leads to new insights or alternative explanations or challenges current understanding (Polit & Beck, 2017). Though case reports can provide the EBP team with insights into a specific clinical situation, they have limited generalizability and, therefore, are Level V evidence. Case reports should not be confused with case studies. Case studies involve a collection of qualitative or quantitative information, may use statistical methods to analyze the data, employ in-depth investigation over time, or study relationships and trends. In these instances, they are considered quantitative, qualitative, or mixed methods research (Sandelowski, 2011).

"A case report is a powerful tool to disseminate information on unusual clinical syndromes, disease associations, unusual side effects to therapy, or response to treatment. Case reports have been used for years as a means to teach health sciences students, and are one of the best ways for authors to get started in scholarly writing, and can be a valuable learning experience for both author and reader. Case reports continue to be a very popular section within the *Journal*. They are well read, and by nature they are easily accessible." (Gopikrishna, 2010)

Community Standard (Level V Evidence)

When an EPB team is searching for evidence, one consideration is the current practice standard in the community. To learn the community standard, the EBP team identifies healthcare providers, agencies, or organizations from which they can gain evidence. The team devises a standard list of questions and a systematic approach to data collection. For example, Johns Hopkins University School of Nursing students were assisting with an EBP project with this question: "Does charge nurse availability during the shift affect staff nurse satisfaction with work flow?" An EBP team member contacted local hospitals to determine whether charge nurses had patient assignments. Students developed a data sheet with questions about the healthcare facility, the unit, the staffing pattern, and staff comments about satisfaction. The students reported the number of units contacted and responses, information source, and number of sources using the Nonresearch Evidence Appraisal Tool. Additionally, this approach provides an opportunity to network with other clinicians about a clinical issue.

Social networking, blogs from a professional organization's websites, and special interest groups are other sources of information about community standards. The online Pediatric Emergency Medicine Database (http://www.pemdatabase.org) provides articles and a discussion list for clinical questions. These types of databases can provide helpful information about community standards.

Clinician Experience (Level V Evidence)

Though this section focuses on nurse experience, the best application of EBP occurs within the interdisciplinary care team because no single discipline provides healthcare in isolation.

The concept of holistic care as the hallmark of nursing expertise, advocated by Benner (2001), supports the notion that evidence of all types (both research and nonresearch) must inform nursing practice. Novice nurses rely heavily on guidelines and care protocols to enhance skill development, looking at the patient as the sum of composite parts. The more experienced expert nurse skillfully synthesizes and applies information from research findings and experience (Garland Baird & Miller, 2015).

Clinical expertise (Level V), both skill proficiency and professional judgment, is gained through the combination of education and clinical experiences. Personal judgments arising from past and present nurse-patient interactions, and knowledge about what works within the organization or system, add depth to that expertise. Nurses who practice within an evidence-based framework are committed to personal growth, reflection, self-evaluation, accountability, and lifelong learning (Dale, 2006).

The Expertise in Practice Project (Hardy, Titchen, Manley, & McCormack, 2006) identified and examined attributes of nurse expertise and enabling factors. Attributes of expertise included:

- **Holistic practice knowledge:** Drawing from a range of knowledge bases to inform action

- **Skilled know-how:** Enabling others by sharing knowledge and skills

- **Saliency:** Observing nonverbal cues to understand each individual's unique situation

- **Moral agency:** Consciously promoting each individual's dignity, respect, and individuality

- **Knowing the patient/client:** Promoting patient decision-making within the context of each individual's unique perspective

Enabling factors for nursing expertise included:

- **Reflectivity:** The ability to continually reconsider, reassess, and reframe one's work

- **Organization of practice:** Organization and prioritization of workload

- **Autonomy and authority:** Taking responsibility for consequences of difficult decisions

- **Good interpersonal relationships:** Being intentional in relationships

- **Recognition from others:** Regular feedback and acknowledgment of work

Patient/Consumer Experience (Level V Evidence)

Patients are consumers of healthcare, and the term *consumer* also refers to a larger group of individuals using health services in a variety of settings. The art of nursing recognizes that humans are active participants in their lives and make choices regarding their health (Milton, 2007). Health is a quality of life and is best described by the person who is experiencing it. Patient experience (Level V) is a core component of a patient-centered approach to care, honoring lived experiences as evidence so that the patient can be an active partner in decision-making. This is based on the core ethical value of respect for persons. Each patient has personal, religious, and cultural beliefs to account for that enable the individual to make informed care decisions. Individuals and families of different cultures, races, social, and economic classes are likely to have quite dissimilar experiences with the healthcare system and, hence, have dissimilar perspectives on EBPs (DelVecchio Good & Hannah, 2015).

The expert nurse incorporates patient preferences into clinical decision-making by asking the following questions:

- Are the research findings and nonresearch evidence relevant to this particular patient's care?

- Have all care and treatment options based on the best available evidence been presented to the patient?

- Has the patient been given as much time as is necessary to allow for clarification and consideration of options?

- Have the patient's expressed preferences and concerns been considered when planning care?

The answer to these questions requires ethical practice and respect for a patient's autonomy. Combining sensitivity to individual patient needs and thoughtful application of best evidence leads to optimal patient-centered outcomes. The Patient-Centered Outcomes Research Institute (PCORI) established by the Affordable Care Act 2010 produces and promotes high-integrity, evidence-based information that comes from research guided by patients, caregivers, and the broader health-care community. This institute is a new source of evidence to guide patients and family preferences for EBP teams.

Patients/consumers play a key role in managing their care. As consumer-driven healthcare has expanded, recent reports recommend specific efforts for consumer education and improving medical literacy (Arblaster, Mackenzie, & Willis, 2015). Nurses are increasingly cognizant of the critical role the consumer plays in the quality and safety of healthcare. Upholding the belief that consumer preferences and values are integral to EBP, Melnyk and Fineout-Overholt (2006) offered three suggestions to involve patients in clinical decision-making: a) respect patient par-ticipation in clinical decision-making, b) assess patient preferences and values dur-ing the admission intake process, and c) provide patient education about treatment plan options. Additionally, providing information to patients about best practice recommendations is important because these apply to their particular clinical situ-ation. Only an informed patient can truly participate in clinical decision-making, ensuring the best possible outcomes of care.

Engaging consumers of healthcare in EBP goes well beyond the individual patient encounter. Consumer organizations can play a significant role in supporting imple-mentation and promulgation of EBP. Consumer-led activities can take the form of facilitating research to expedite equitable adoption of new and existing best prac-tices, promoting policies for the development and use of advocacy toolkits, and influencing provider adoption of EBP (DelVecchio Good & Hannah, 2015). In ex-amining the information provided by consumers, the EBP team should consider the credibility of the individual or group. What segment and volume of the consumer group do they represent? Do their comments and opinions provide any insight into your EBP question?

An EBP team should consider the perspectives of children, young families, the elderly, and aging families. They should ascertain whether suggested recommenda-tions have been designed and developed with sensitivity and knowledge of diverse cultural groups.

Recommendations for Nurse Leaders

Time and resource constraints compel nurse leaders to find creative ways to support integration of new knowledge into clinical practice. The amount of time the average staff nurse has to devote to gathering and appraising evidence is limited. Therefore, finding the most efficient way to gain new knowledge should be a goal of EBP initiatives (Chapter 9 suggests ways to build organizational EBP infrastructure). Nurse leaders should not only support staff education initiatives that teach nurses how to read and interpret evidence but also become familiar themselves with desired attributes of such reviews so that they can serve as credible mentors in the change process.

The challenge to the nurse is to combine the contributions of the two evidence types (research and nonresearch) in making patient care decisions. According to Melnyk and Fineout-Overholt (2006), no "magic bullet" or standard formula exists with which to determine how much weight should be applied to each of these factors when making patient care decisions. It is not sufficient to apply a standard rating system that grades the level and quality of evidence without determining whether recommendations made by the best evidence are compatible with the patient's values and preferences and the clinician's expertise. Nurse leaders can best support EBP by providing clinicians with the knowledge and skills necessary to appraise quantitative and qualitative research evidence within the context of nonresearch evidence. Only through continuous learning can clinicians gain the confidence needed to incorporate the broad range of evidence into the more targeted care of individual patients.

Summary

This chapter describes nonresearch evidence and strategies for evaluating this evidence and recommends approaches for building nurses' capacity to appraise nonresearch evidence to inform their practice. Nonresearch evidence includes summaries of evidence (clinical practice guidelines, consensus or position statements, literature and integrative reviews); organizational experience (quality improvement and financial data); expert opinion (individual commentary or opinion, case reports); community standards; clinician experience; and consumer experience.

This evidence includes important information for practice decision. For example, consumer preference is an essential element of the EBP process with increased focus on patient-centered care. In summary, though nonresearch evidence does not have the rigor of research evidence, it does provide important information for informed practice decisions.

References

The AGREE Research Trust. (2013). The AGREE II instrument. Retrieved from http://www.agreetrust.org/wp-content/uploads/2013/10/AGREE-II-Users-Manual-and-23-item-Instrument_2009_UPDATE_2013.pdf

Arblaster, K., Mackenzie, L., & Willis, K. (2015). Mental health consumer participation in education: A structured literature review. *Australian Occupational Therapy Journal, 62*(5), 341–362. doi:10.1111/1440-1630.12205

Arveklev, S. H., Wigert, H., Berg, L., Burton, B., & Lepp, M. (2015). The use and application of drama in nursing education—An integrative review of the literature. *Nurse Education Today, 35*(7), e12–e17. doi:http://dx.doi.org/10.1016/j.nedt.2015.02.025

Benner, P. E. (2001). *From novice to expert: Excellence and power in clinical nursing practice* (Commemorative ed.). Upper Saddle River, NJ: Prentice Hall.

Black, A. E., Flynn, P. E. R., Smith, H. L., Thomas, M. L., & Wilkinson, K. A. (2015). Development of a guideline for the management of the unanticipated difficult airway in pediatric practice. *Pediatric Anesthesia, 25*(4), 346–362. doi:10.1111/pan.12615

Brouwers, M. C., Kho, M. E., Browman, G. P., Burgers, J. S., Cluzeau, F., Feder, G., Fervers, B., Graham, I. D., Hanna, S. E., & Makarski, J. (2010). Development of the AGREE II, part 1: Performance, usefulness and areas for improvement. *Canadian Medical Association Journal, 182*(10), 1045–1062.

Carande-Kulis, V. G., Maciosek, M. V., Briss, P. A., Teutsch, S. M., Zaza, S., Truman, B. I.,...Task Force on Community Preventive Services. (2000). Methods for systematic reviews of economic evaluations for the guide to community preventive service. *American Journal of Preventive Medicine, 18*(1S), 75–91.

Carper, B. (1978). Fundamental patterns of knowing in nursing. *ANS Advances in Nursing Science, 1*(1), 13–23.

Centers for Disease Control and Prevention (CDC). (2007). Economic evaluation of public health preparedness and response efforts. Retrieved from http://www.cdc.gov/owcd/EET/SeriesIntroduction/TOC.html

Cohen, R. I., Kennedy, H., Amitrano, B., Dillon, M., Guigui, S., & Kanner, A. (2015). A quality improvement project to decrease emergency department and medical intensive care unit transfer times. *Journal of Critical Care, 30*(6), 1331–1337. doi:http://dx.doi.org/10.1016/j.jcrc.2015.07.017

Community guide economic evaluation abstraction form, Version 4.0. (2010). Retrieved from http://www.thecommunityguide.org/about/EconAbstraction_v5.pdf

Conn, V. S. (2004). Meta-analysis research. *Journal of Vascular Nursing, 22*(2), 51–52.

Dale, A. E. (2006). Determining guiding principles for evidence-based practice. *Nursing Standard, 20*(25), 41–46.

Dans, A. M., Dans, L., Oxman, A. D., Robinson, V., Acuin, J., Tugwell, P., … Kang, D. (2007). Assessing equity in clinical practice guidelines. *Journal of Clinical Epidemiology, 60*(6), 540–546.

DelVecchio Good, M.-J., & Hannah, S. D. (2015). "Shattering culture": Perspectives on cultural competence and evidence-based practice in mental health services. *Transcultural Psychiatry, 52*(2), 198–221. doi:10.1177/1363461514557348

Deresinski, S., & File, T. M., Jr. (2011). Improving clinical practice guidelines—The answer is more clinical research. *Archives of Internal Medicine, 171*(15), 1402–1403.

Fervers, B., Burgers, J. S., Haugh, M. C., Brouwers, M., Browman, G., Cluzeau, F., & Philip, T. (2005). Predictors of high quality clinical practice guidelines: Examples in oncology. *International Journal for Quality in Health Care, 17*(2), 123–132.

Garland Baird, L. M., & Miller, T. (2015). Factors influencing evidence-based practice for community nurses. *British Journal of Community Nursing, 20*(5), 233–242. doi:10.12968/bjcn.2015.20.5.233

Gopikrishna, V. (2010). A report on case reports. *Journal of Conservative Dentistry, 13*(4): 265–271. doi: 10.4103/0972-0707.73375

Grant, M. J., & Booth, A. (2009). A typology of reviews: An analysis of 14 review types and associated methodologies. *Health Information and Libraries Journal, 26*(2), 91–108.

Hardy, S., Titchen, A., Manley, K., & McCormack, B. (2006). Re-defining nursing expertise in the United Kingdom. *Nursing Science Quarterly, 19*(3), 260–264.

Institute for Healthcare Improvement (IHI). (2013). STate Action on Avoidable Rehospitalizations (STAAR) initiative. Retrieved from http://www.ihi.org/offerings/Initiatives/STAAR/Pages/GetInvolved.aspx

Institute of Medicine (IOM). (1992). *Guidelines for clinical practice: From development to use.* In M. J. Field & K. N. Lohr (Eds.). Washington, DC: National Academy Press.

Institute of Medicine (IOM). (2001). *Crossing the quality chasm: A new health system for the 21st century.* Washington, DC: National Academy Press.

Institute of Medicine (IOM). (2011). *Clinical practice guidelines we can trust.* Retrieved from http://www.nationalacademies.org/hmd/Reports/2011/Clinical-Practice-Guidelines-We-Can-Trust/Standards.aspx

Joussemet, M., Mageau, G. A., & Koestner, R. (2014). Promoting optimal parenting and children's mental health: A preliminary evaluation of the how-to parenting program. *Journal of Child and Family Studies, 23*(6), 949–964. doi:10.1007/s10826-013-9751-0

Kuehn, B. M. (2011). IOM sets out "gold standard" practices for creating guidelines, systematic reviews. *JAMA, 305*(18), 1846–1848.

Lopez-Olivo, M. A., Kallen, M. A., Ortiz, Z., Skidmore, B., & Suarez-Almazor, M. E. (2008). Quality appraisal of clinical practice guidelines and consensus statements on the use of biologic agents in rheumatoid arthritis: A systematic review. *Arthritis & Rheumatism, 59*(11), 1625–1638.

Melnyk, B. M., & Fineout-Overholt, E. (2006). Consumer preferences and values as an integral key to evidence-based practice. *Nursing Administration Quarterly, 30*(2), 123–127.

Milton, C. (2007). Evidence-based practice: Ethical questions for nursing. *Nursing Science Quarterly, 20*(2), 123–126.

Mims, J. W. (2015). Targeting quality improvement in clinical practice guidelines. *Otolaryngology— Head and Neck Surgery: Official Journal of American Academy of Otolaryngology—Head and Neck Surgery, 153*(6), 907–908. doi:10.1177/0194599815611861

National Guideline Clearinghouse (NGC). (2013). Criteria for inclusion of clinical practice guidelines in NGC. Retrieved from https://www.guideline.gov/help-and-about/summaries/inclusion-criteria

Netherwood, M., Skittrall, R., & Alexis, O. (2014). Regulation of nursing assistants: A critical international issue? *Contemporary Nurse: A Journal for the Australian Nursing Profession, 48*(2), 197–198. doi:10.5172/conu.2014.48.2.197

Newhouse, R. P., Pettit, J. C., Poe, S., & Rocco, L. (2006). The slippery slope: Differentiating between quality improvement and research. *Journal of Nursing Administration, 36*(4), 211–219.

Ogrinc, G., Davies, L., Batalden, P., Davidoff, F., Goodman, D., & Stevens, D. (2015). SQUIRE 2.0. Retrieved from http://www.squire-statement.org

Patient-Centered Outcomes Research Institute. (n.d.). Our mission. Retrieved from http://www.pcori.org

Polit, D. F., & Beck, C. T. (2017). *Nursing Research: Generating and assessing evidence for nursing practice* (9th ed.). Philadelphia, PA: Wolters Kluwer Lippincott Williams & Wilkins.

Sandelowski, M. (2011). "Casing" the research case study. *Research in Nursing & Health, 34*, 153–159.

Scala, E., Price, C., & Day, D. (2016). An integrative review of engaging clinical nurses in nursing research. *Journal of Nursing Scholarship, 48*(4), 423–430.

Shiffman, R. N., Shekelle, P., Overhage, M., Slutsky, J., Grimshaw, J., & Deshpande, A. M. (2003). Standardized reporting of clinical practice guidelines: A proposal from the conference on guideline standardization. *Annals of Internal Medicine, 139*(6), 493–498.

Spetz, J., Brown, D. S., Aydin, C., & Donaldson, N. (2013). The value of reducing hospital-acquired pressure ulcer prevalence: An illustrative analysis. *Journal of Nursing Administration, 43*(4), 235–241.

Stetler, C. B., Morsi, D., Rucki, S., Broughton, S., Corrigan, B., Fitzgerald, J.,…Sheridan, E. A. (1998). Utilization-focused integrative reviews in a nursing service. *Applied Nursing Research, 11*(4), 195–206.

Stone, N. J., Robinson, J. G., Lichtenstein, A. H., Bairey Merz, C. N., Blum, C. B., Eckel, R. H., Wilson, P. W. F. (2014). 2013 ACC/AHA Guideline on the treatment of blood cholesterol to reduce atherosclerotic cardiovascular risk in adults. A Report of the American College of Cardiology/American Heart Association Task Force on Practice Guidelines. *Journal of the American College of Cardiology, 63*(25, Part B), 2889–2934. doi:http://dx.doi.org/10.1016/j.jacc.2013.11.002

Whittemore, R. (2005). Combining evidence in nursing research: Methods and implications. *Nursing Research, 54*(1), 56–62.

Whittemore, R., & Knafl, K. (2005). The integrative review: Updated methodology. *Journal of Advanced Nursing, 52*(5), 546–553.

Yang, P. H., Hung, C. H., & Chen, Y. C. (2015). The impact of three nursing staffing models on nursing outcomes. *Journal of Advanced Nursing, 71*(8), 1847–1856. doi:10.1111/jan.12643

Yoder-Wise, P. S. (2014). *Leading and managing in nursing* (6th ed.). St. Louis, MO: Mosby.

Translation

The final phase of the Practice question, Evidence, Translation (PET) process is *translation*, which assesses the recommendations identified in the evidence phase for transferability to a desired practice setting. If appropriate, the practices are implemented, evaluated, and communicated both within and outside the organization. Translation is the value-added step in evidence-based practice, leading to a change in practice (EBP), processes, or systems and in resulting outcomes. This chapter covers the translation phase of the PET process, which includes the practice decision, implementation, and dissemination. This chapter:

- Examines criteria that determine recommendation for implementation

- Distinguishes among EBP, research, and quality improvement (QI)

- Specifies the components of an action plan

- Identifies steps in implementing change

- Describes potential forums for communicating results

Translation is the primary reason to conduct an evidence-based review. Paying particular attention to the planning and implementation of recommendations can improve the potential for successfully meeting the project's goals. Additionally, fully realized translation requires organizational resources and commitment. Critically appraising, rating, and grading the evidence and making practice recommendations requires one set of skills; translation requires another. Change theory, motivational theory, political and power dynamics, and organizational processes are activated during translation.

Translation Models

There is still much to learn about evidence translation. What is known is that translation should be a) based on synthesis of research results tailored to the specific stakeholders to which the evidence translation is targeted and b) informed by a baseline assessment of contextual barriers and facilitators encountered (Grimshaw, Eccles, Lavis, Hill, & Squires, 2012).

The use of a model or framework for translation is important in ensuring a systematic approach to the change. First and foremost, fully realized translation requires organizational support, human and material resources, and a commitment of individuals and interprofessional teams. Context, communication, leadership, mentoring, and evidence matter for the implementation and dissemination of new knowledge into practice. Planning and active coordination by the EBP team are critical to successful translation of evidence into practice, as are adherence to principles of change that guide this process and careful attention to the characteristics of the organization involved (Newhouse, 2007a; White, Dudley-Brown, and Terhaar, 2016).

We will describe three models that have been used by nurses: Knowledge to Action (KTA), Promoting Action on Research Implementation in Health Services (PARIHS), and the Translation Research Model.

The University of Ottawa's KTA model uses the word *action* rather than *practice* because it is intended for a wider range of knowledge users and not just clinicians (Graham, Tetroe, & KT Theories Research Group, 2007). The KTA process includes these steps:

1. Identify a problem for review.

2. Adapt new knowledge to the local context.

3. Assess barriers to use.

4. Select, tailor, and implement interventions to promote the knowledge.

5. Monitor its use.

6. Evaluate the outcomes.

7. Ensure sustainability in practice (Canadian Institute of Health Research, 2016).

The PARIHS model, used widely in nursing, identifies essential determinants of successful implementation of research into clinical practice. The three core elements are the nature of the *evidence*, the quality of the *context* or the environment in which the implementation will occur, and the strategies for *facilitation* of the translation of evidence into practice (Kitson et al., 2008). The central role of facilitation in evidence translation engages team members in the change and appreciates the context in which the change occurs (Kitson & Harvey, 2016). Facilitator skill and experience range from novice to expert, with complex projects requiring expertise in implementation methods.

Finally, the Translation Research Model (Titler, 2010; Titler & Everett, 2001), which is built on the important diffusion of innovations work by Everett Rogers (2003), provides a framework for selecting strategies to promote adoption of EBPs. According to this framework, adoption of new evidence into practice is influenced by the type and strength of the evidence, the communication or dissemination plan, the clinicians, and the characteristics of the organization.

Requirements for Successful Translation

In the past, evidence known to affect successful translation has often not been implemented or has been implemented inconsistently. As the quest to improve the quality of healthcare has increased in importance, evidence translation has achieved a higher priority. In addition, better systematic implementation strategies and frameworks have been developed to escalate the translation process and ensure success.

When planning for evidence translation, the final step in the PET process, follow these steps (see Appendix A):

- Determine the fit, feasibility, and appropriateness of recommendations for the translation path.
- Create the action plan.
- Secure support and resources to implement the action plan.
- Implement the action plan.
- Evaluate the outcomes.
- Report the outcomes to stakeholders.
- Identify the next steps.
- Disseminate the findings.

Path to Translation

The evidence phase of the PET process ends when the team develops recommendations based on the synthesis of findings and strength of the evidence. The JHNEBP Model has four possible paths for translating evidence into practice, based on the type of available evidence:

- Strong, compelling evidence, consistent results
- Good evidence, consistent results
- Good evidence but conflicting results
- Insufficient or absent evidence

Strong, compelling evidence, consistent results: When strong, compelling evidence is available, the application to practice is quite clear, particularly if the evidence includes several Level I research studies. For example, it is easy to recommend a practice change if you have three, high-quality, randomized, controlled trials with consistent results or if there is a meta-analysis (Level I) related to the question. However, this is not often the case with nursing questions.

Good evidence, consistent results. In many cases, the EBP team encounters good overall evidence yielding consistent findings across studies, but the design and quality may vary. There may be concerns about control of bias (i.e., internal and external validity); adequate comparisons; or study design and methods for which conclusions cannot be drawn. For example, the team may find only non-experimental studies without comparison groups or only descriptive correlational surveys, or the evidence may include multiple study designs such as quasi-experimental, nonexperimental, and expert opinion. In these circumstances, and particularly in the absence of Level I evidence, evaluation of the potential risks and benefits is in order before recommending a change in practice. If the benefits outweigh the risks, the EBP team should develop a pilot to test any practice change and evaluate outcomes prior to full-scale implementation.

Good evidence, but conflicting results. In this situation, the overall evidence summary includes studies with conflicting findings. Such evidence is difficult to interpret. When this is the case, undertaking a practice change cannot be recommended. The EBP team may decide to review the literature periodically for new evidence to answer the question or perhaps to conduct their own research study.

Insufficient or absent evidence. Where little or no evidence exists in the public domain to answer the EBP question, the team cannot recommend a practice change. The team may decide to search for new evidence periodically, design their own research study, or cancel the project entirely.

Determine Fit, Feasibility, and Appropriateness of Recommendation(s) for Translation

Practice recommendations made in the evidence phase, even if based on strong evidence, cannot be implemented in all settings. The EBP team is responsible for determining the fit, feasibility, and appropriateness of the recommendations for translation (see Appendix H). These are the main questions to be considered: Can this practice change be implemented given the current organizational infrastructure? What additional actions or resources are needed? Specific criteria can be helpful to make this determination. Stetler (2001, 2010) recommends using the criteria of *substantiating evidence*, *fit of setting*, *feasibility*, and *current practice*.

When considering the overall evidence summary, the team should assess the finding's *consistency* (whether results were the same in the other evidence reviewed), *quality* or *applicability* (the extent to which bias was minimized in individual studies so that the evidence is generalizable to the population or setting of interest), and *quantity* (number, sample size and power, and size of effect; Agency for Healthcare Research and Quality, 2002; White et al., 2016).

Organizational context and infrastructure such as resources (equipment or products), change agency (linkages with people who foster change or adoption of evidence), and organizational readiness also need to be considered (Greenhalgh, Robert, Bate, Macfarlane, & Kyriakidou, 2005). Additionally, nursing-related factors such as nursing processes, policies, and competencies need to be present before implementing recommendations. The following guiding questions can help to determine whether the proposed recommendation adds value:

- Would this change improve clinical outcomes?

- Would this change improve patient or nurse satisfaction?

- Would this change reduce the cost of care for patients?

- Would this change improve unit operations?

Determining the feasibility of implementing EBP recommendations is essential in assessing whether they add significant value to improving a specific problem. Implementing processes with a low likelihood of success wastes valuable time and resources on efforts that produce negligible benefits.

The team should also assess the system's readiness for change and determine strategies to overcome possible barriers to implementation. Readiness for change includes the availability of human and material resources, current processes, support from decision-makers (individuals and groups), and budget implications. Implementation strategies include communication and education plans and involvement of stakeholders and other individuals affected by the change.

Evidence-Based Practice, Research, and QI

Although a discussion of how to conduct research to test a new procedure or product is beyond the scope of this chapter, it is important to clearly differentiate the activities of research, QI, and EBP (Newhouse, 2007b; Newhouse, Pettit, Poe, & Rocco, 2006; Shirey et al., 2011). Box 8.1 provides the common definitions and an example of each. Note that research requires additional organizational infrastructure, including affiliation with an institutional review board (IRB), experienced mentors who can serve as principal investigators, education in human subject research, and a number of additional research competencies.

Box 8.1   Differentiating EBP, Quality Improvement, and Research

EBP

The EBP process identifies, appraises, and uses existing high-quality research and nonresearch evidence to identify best practice to drive practice improvements.

EBP Example: For adult patients admitted with heart failure who smoke, what is the best strategy to improve the success of quit attempts? An evidence review is conducted using the PET process, and recommendations are generated. These are implemented and then evaluated using the QI process.

Quality Improvement

QI focus is a local unit or organization improvement effort that uses small tests of change and monitors effectiveness of change. Models such as PDSA and DEMAC are often used as guides for implementing a QI process.

In QI, teams use systematic and continuous actions toward healthcare service improvements to systems and processes with the intent to improve the health of patients (Health Resources Services Administration, 2016). QI results are often

continues

> **Box 8.1   Differentiating EBP, Quality Improvement, and Research (continued)**
>
> disseminated outside the organization in the form of lessons learned, but they are not generalizable beyond the organization. In certain situations, however, the goal of the activity is to not only improve care but also generalize knowledge for research purposes. In these cases, it is important to determine whether the regulations that relate to protection of human subjects apply (U.S. Department of Health and Human Services, 2016a, 2016b). http://www.hhs.gov/ohrp/regulations-and-policy/guidance/faq/Quality-Improvement-Activities/index.html
>
> http://www.hhs.gov/ohrp/regulations-and-policy/decision-charts/index.html
>
> QI Example: Review medical records to assess whether guideline-based smoking cessation counseling is used for patients with heart failure in a specific unit or organization. Compliance with the smoking cessation standard is measured as present or absent for patients and is reported for improvement purposes and public information.
>
> **Research**
>
> Research generates new knowledge and is "a systematic investigation, including research development, testing, and evaluation, designed to develop or contribute to generalizable knowledge" (U.S. Department of Health and Human Services, 2009, 45 CFR 46.102[d]). Research activities are intended to be generalized or applied outside an organization and require compliance with Office for Human Research Protections (OHRP) regulations and, sometimes, the Food and Drug Administration (FDA).
>
> Research Examples: A randomized cluster design is used to test whether a quality collaborative improves the quality of smoking cessation counseling for people admitted to the hospital with heart failure who smoke (Newhouse et al., 2013).

Create an Action Plan for Translation

Creating an action plan provides manageable steps to implement change and assigns responsibility for carrying the project forward. The EBP team develops specific change strategies to introduce, promote, and evaluate the practice change. It can be helpful to formulate the plan in a template that includes a timeline with progress columns (see Appendix I).

The action plan includes:

- Development of (or a change to) a protocol, guideline, critical path, system, or process related to the EBP question

- Specification of a detailed timeline, assignment of team members to tasks, an evaluation process, and a plan for how results will be reported
- Solicitation of feedback on the action plan from organizational leadership, bedside clinicians, and other stakeholders

The action plan begins with an organizational assessment to evaluate the readiness of the organization or the context for change. Organizational infrastructure is the cornerstone of successful translation (Newhouse, 2010b). Infrastructure provides human and material resources that are fundamental in preparation for change (Greenhalgh et al., 2005; Newhouse, 2007a). Organizational readiness is leveraged by assessing the current state and strategically planning for building the capacity of the organization before implementation can begin.

Beyond human and material readiness, teams also need to consider organizational culture. *Organizational culture* refers to group-learned assumptions as the organization integrates and adapts to external forces. These assumptions become an attribute of the group and are then taught as the right way to "perceive, think, and feel in relation to problems" (Schein, 2004, p. 17). To change the culture, the team must challenge tradition, reinforce the need for evidence to drive decisions, and change old patterns of behavior, which sometimes requires new skills in evidence review. Additional detail and tools to assess organizational readiness and culture are available elsewhere (Newhouse, 2010a).

Ensure Successful Action Planning

To ensure a successful translation (see Appendix A), first appoint a project leader and identify change champions who are supportive of the recommended practice change and who will be able to support the project leader during the translation phase of the project. Once this leader is identified and change champions are on board, consider whether the translation activities will require any additional skills, knowledge, or particular individuals who can assist with or will be essential to the success of the work. These additional members, often referred to as *opinion leaders,* are usually well-known individuals to the practice group in the organization who are held in high esteem and could influence the practice group's opinion for or against the change. The opinion leader is often someone that the group members turn to for advice, opinions, or views on matters of importance, so it is critical to identify them in the process.

Once this group is organized, its members identify barriers and facilitators to the success of the proposed practice change, identifying strengths that can be leveraged to overcome the barriers. They would also discuss how the change will impact current policies and procedures, the workflow and throughput of the unit or department, and technological supports to the group's usual work, such as the electronic health record (EHR) or another technology that the group depends on.

Identify Milestones and Critical Tasks

The action plan should include the identification of critical milestones and other essential tasks to be completed for the translation. The milestones should include a schedule of all necessary activities, with an assignment of who is responsible for each activity and the target time frame for completion. The action plan should also include activities associated with collection and analysis of the pre- and post-measures for evaluation of the practice change (see Appendix B).

Secure and Confirm Support and Availability of Resources

Securing support from stakeholders and decision-makers is critical to the implementation of recommendations. Availability of funds to cover expenses associated with the translation and the allocation of human, material, and technological resources is dependent on the endorsement of stakeholders such as organizational leaders or committees and in collaboration with those individuals or groups affected by the recommendations. For success, it may also be necessary to bring in content or external experts to consult on the translation. The cost of these resources should be estimated and budgeted and an implementation plan formulated. Decision-makers may support wide implementation of the change, request a small test of the change to validate results, revise the plan or recommendations, or reject the implementation plan. Preparing for the presentation or meeting with decision-makers, involving stakeholders (see Appendix C), and creating a comprehensive implementation plan are the key steps in building organizational support. Finally, estimation of and feasibility to secure dissemination costs, such as travel and other costs associated with presentation or poster development, should be discussed.

Implement the Action Plan

After an action plan is created and support is secured, implementation begins. The first step is a small test of the change, or *pilot*. The implementation plan is communicated to all team members who are affected by the change or who are caring for a patient or population affected by the change. This communication can take the form of an agenda item at a staff meeting, an inservice, a direct mailing, an email, a bulletin board, or a video, for example. Team members must know who the project leader is, where to access needed information or supplies, and how to communicate to the project leader any issues as they arise. The team obtains staff input along the way to identify problems and address them as soon as possible. Changes are then implemented and evaluated.

Evaluate Outcomes

After the change is implemented, the next step is to evaluate its impact and progress toward the desired outcomes. Outcomes identified when formulating the PICO are the measures used to evaluate the success of the change. Collaborating with the organization's QI staff is important during the evaluation process for guidance on the tools and the appropriate intervals to measure the change. Selecting and developing outcome measures includes defining the purpose of measurement, choosing the clinical areas to evaluate, selecting and developing the metrics, and evaluating the results (Pronovost, Miller, Dorman, Berenholtz, & Rubin, 2001 [adapted from McGlynn, 1998]). Measures may include *process measures* (focus on steps in the system), *outcome measures* (focus on results of system performance), or *balancing measures* (focus on impact on other parts of the system) (Institute for Healthcare Improvement, 2011). Data collected are compared to baseline data to determine whether the change should be implemented on a wider scale. Descriptive data, such as *frequencies* or *means,* can be graphically displayed in bar, line, or run charts.

Report Outcomes to Stakeholders

After the outcome evaluation, the team should follow up with a report to the appropriate committee or decision-makers. Decision-makers can be members of a committee, such as a research or quality improvement committee, or organizational leaders. In reporting the outcomes to stakeholders, carefully consider the initial problem, the recommended practice change, and the project findings. What is the most important information that needs to be conveyed to the stakeholder group? What are the key messages? These messages should be aligned to the stakeholder audience. For example, your presentation to the interprofessional stakeholder group may differ from the key messages communicated to departmental leadership (see Appendix J). The report should be a succinct communication, in executive summary format, and consistent with organizational templates. Box 8.2 provides an example of an executive summary framed in the PET template.

Box 8.2   Example of Template for Executive Summary Using PET

Problem

There is an increase in the incidence of postoperative pressure ulcers. When patients are positioned in the operating room, the team uses multiple positioning aids, and no standard exists for positioning based on the type of surgery.

Practice Question

What are the most effective interventions to prevent skin pressure in adult patients undergoing surgery?

Evidence

CINAHL and PubMed were searched using the keywords *perioperative* or *surgery,* AND *positioning,* AND *pressure ulcers;* 18 sources of evidence were reviewed (see the following table).

Box 8.2   Example of Template for Executive Summary Using PET (continued)

Level Type	Number of Sources	Overall Quality Rating	Synthesis of Findings (Evidence That Answers the EBP Question)
Level I	5	B	■ Foam is not found to be better than conventional nursing care. ■ Gel pads are better than standard operating room (OR) mattresses. ■ Screening should be conducted for specific risk factors. ■ There is no difference between low-flow-pressure mattresses and alternating-pressure mattresses. ■ Multicell dynamic-pressure pulsating mattresses are more effective than conventional mattresses.
Level II	4	B	■ Conduct screening for specific risk factors. ■ Alternating-pressure systems are effective. ■ Viscoelastic polyether is more effective than foam or gel.
Level III	2	A–B	■ Screening should be conducted for specific risk factors.
Level IV	0		
Level V	7	B	■ Fluid pad reduces pressure ulcers. ■ Foam overlays have the lowest pressure reduction. ■ Gel pads allow for some pressure reduction. ■ Dynamic-air-pressure mattresses are promising but need more research. ■ Foam pads are not effective in reducing capillary interface pressure because they quickly compress under heavy body areas. ■ Use of gel pads or similar devices over the OR bed decreases pressure at any given point by redistributing overall pressure across a larger surface area. ■ Foam mattress overlays are effective in reducing pressure only if they are made of thick and dense foam that resists compression. ■ Pillows, blankets, and molded foam devices produce only a minimum of pressure reduction. ■ Towels and sheet rolls do not reduce pressure and may contribute to friction injuries.

continues

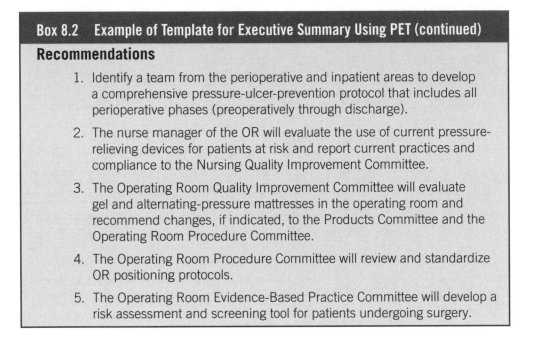

Box 8.2   Example of Template for Executive Summary Using PET (continued)

Recommendations

1. Identify a team from the perioperative and inpatient areas to develop a comprehensive pressure-ulcer-prevention protocol that includes all perioperative phases (preoperatively through discharge).

2. The nurse manager of the OR will evaluate the use of current pressure-relieving devices for patients at risk and report current practices and compliance to the Nursing Quality Improvement Committee.

3. The Operating Room Quality Improvement Committee will evaluate gel and alternating-pressure mattresses in the operating room and recommend changes, if indicated, to the Products Committee and the Operating Room Procedure Committee.

4. The Operating Room Procedure Committee will review and standardize OR positioning protocols.

5. The Operating Room Evidence-Based Practice Committee will develop a risk assessment and screening tool for patients undergoing surgery.

Identify Next Steps

After the successful implementation and favorable evaluation of recommendations, and with support from decision-makers, changes are implemented on a wider scale, if appropriate. The team reviews the process and results and considers the next steps. Organization-wide, or additional unit implementation, requires a modified action plan and, possibly, reassignment of responsibilities to an individual, a team, or a committee. Considerations for the new team can include a new question that emerges from the process, additional training or education for colleagues involved in the process change, and suggestions for new measures or tools for the evaluation. The recommendations are then implemented and evaluated.

Disseminate Findings

The level of communication regarding the findings and dissemination of information is based on the scope and complexity of the problem. Evidence-based project outcomes are communicated internally to all members involved in the care of the patient or population affected by the practice changes. This communication can take the form of committees or conferences, internal meetings, publications in newsletters, or the intranet.

Additionally, it may be appropriate to present results at professional conferences or in suitable EBP publications, sharing lessons learned, actions that worked, actions that did not, or the resulting clinical and fiscal outcomes, for example. Methods of external dissemination may also include podium or poster presentations, publication in electronic media, or publication in journals whose focus is quality improvement.

Specific guidance on how to develop abstracts, presentations, and publications is available (Krenzischek & Newhouse, 2005). Attending presentations at local, national, and international professional organizations or university conferences is an excellent way to gain presentation experience. See Table 8.1 for links to general and specialty organization websites. Search each website for appropriate conferences, dates, and locations, and communicate the opportunity via electronic media such as group email, or the organization's intranet. Announcements of upcoming conferences generally include information about calls for abstracts; each abstract has specific instructions for content, length, and responsibilities.

Table 8.1   Websites for Potential Conferences to Present EBP Projects

Organization	Website
Sigma Theta Tau International	http://www.nursingsociety.org
American Nurses Association	http://www.nursingworld.org/MainMenuCategories/Conference
American Nurses Association Specialty Nursing Practice Links	http://www.nursingworld.org/EspeciallyForYou/Links/SpecialtyNursing.aspx
American Nurses Credentialing Center National Magnet Conference	http://www.nursecredentialing.org/Magnet/MagnetEvents.aspx

Many professional nursing and multidisciplinary journals and newsletters publish manuscripts about EBP projects. Author guidelines are usually available via the Internet for review. *Worldviews on Evidence-Based Nursing* focuses specifically on EBP and is an excellent resource for a potential publication.

Summary

Translation is the outcome of the PET process. The PET process is linear, but many steps in the process can generate new questions, recommendations, or actions. The organizational infrastructure needed to foster translation includes budgetary support; human and material resources; and the commitment of individuals, stakeholders, and interprofessional teams. Translation is the essence of the EBP process and the cornerstone of best practice. Translation of recommendations requires organizational skills, project management, and leaders with a high level of influence and tenacity—the perfect job for nurses.

References

Agency for Healthcare Research and Quality. (2002). Systems to rate the strength of scientific evidence. *Summary, Evidence Report/Technology Assessment: Number 47* (Rep. No. 02-E015). Rockville, MD. Available at http://archive.ahrq.gov/clinic/epcsums/strengthsum.htm

Canadian Institute of Health Research. (2016). The knowledge to action cycle. Available at http://ktclearinghouse.ca/knowledgebase/knowledgetoaction

Graham, I., Tetroe, J., KT Theories Research Group. (2007). Some theoretical underpinnings of knowledge translation. *Academic Emergency Medicine, 14*(11), 936–941.

Greenhalgh, T., Robert, G., Bate, P., Macfarlane, A., & Kyriakidou, O. (2005). Diffusion of innovations in health service organizations: A systematic literature review. Massachusetts: Blackwell Publishing Ltd.

Grimshaw, J. M., Eccles, M. P., Lavis, J. N., Hill, S. J., & Squires, J. E. (2012). Knowledge translation of research findings. *Implementation Science, 7* (50). doi: 10.1186/1748-5908-7-50

Health Resources Services Administration. (2016). Quality improvement. Available at http://www.hrsa.gov/quality/toolbox/methodology/qualityimprovement

Institute for Healthcare Improvement. (2011). Science of improvement: Establishing measures. Retrieved from http://www.ihi.org/knowledge/Pages/HowtoImprove/ScienceofImprovementEstablishingMeasures.aspx

Kitson, A., & Harvey, G. (2016). Methods to succeed in effective knowledge translation in clinical practice. *Journal of Nursing Scholarship, 48*(3), 294–302. doi:10.1111/jnu.12206

Kitson, A., Rycroft-Malone, J., Harvey, G., McCormack, B., Seers, K., & Titchen, A. (2008). Evaluating the successful implementation of evidence into practice using the PARiHS framework: theoretical and practical challenges. *Implementation Science, 3*(1). Retrieved from http://www.implementationscience.com/content/pdf/1748-5908-3-1.pdf

Krenzischek, D. A., Newhouse, R. (2005). Dissemination of findings. In R. Newhouse & S. Poe (Eds.), *Measuring patient safety* (pp. 67–78). Boston: Jones and Bartlett Publishers.

McGlynn, E. A. (1998). Choosing and evaluating clinical performance measures. *Joint Commission Journal of Quality Improvement, 24*(9), 470–479.

Newhouse, R. P. (2007a). Creating infrastructure supportive of evidence-based nursing practice: leadership strategies. *Worldviews on Evidence-Based Nursing, 4*(1), 21–29.

Newhouse, R. P. (2007b). Diffusing confusion among evidence-based practice, quality improvement, and research. *Journal of Nursing Administration, 37*(10), 432–435.

Newhouse, R. P. (2010a). Instruments to assess organizational readiness for evidence-based practice. *Journal of Nursing Administration, 40*(10), 404–407.

Newhouse, R. P. (2010b). Establishing organizational infrastructure. In S. S. Poe and K. M. White (Eds.), *Johns Hopkins Nursing Evidence-Based Practice Implementation and Translation* (pp. 55–72). Sigma Theta Tau International: Indianapolis, IN.

Newhouse, R. P., Dennison-Himmelfarb, C., Morlock, L., Frick, K., Pronovost, P., & Liang, Y. (2013). A cluster randomized trial of rural hospitals testing a quality collaborative to improve heart failure care: organizational context matters. *Medical Care, 51*(5), 396–403. doi: 10.1097/MLR.0b013e318286e32e

Newhouse, R. P., Pettit, J. C., Poe, S., & Rocco, L. (2006). The slippery slope: Differentiating between quality improvement and research. *Journal of Nursing Administration, 36*(4), 211–219.

Pronovost, P. J., Miller, M. R., Dorman, T., Berenholtz, S. M., & Rubin, H. (2001). Developing and implementing measures of quality of care in the intensive care unit. *Current Opinion in Critical Care, 7*(4), 297–303.

Rogers, E. M. (2003). *Diffusion of innovations* (5th ed.). New York: Free Press.

Schein, E. H. (2004). *Organizational culture and leadership* (3rd ed.). San Francisco: Jossey-Bass.

Shirey, M. R., Hauck, S. L., Embree, J. L., Kinner, T. J., Schaar, G. L., Phillips, L. A., Ashby, S. R., Swenty, C. F., McCool, I. A. (2011). Showcasing differences between quality improvement, evidence-based practice, and research. *Journal of Continuing Education in Nursing, 42*(2), 57–68.

Stetler, C. B. (2001). Updating the Stetler Model of research utilization to facilitate evidence-based practice. *Nursing Outlook, 49*(6), 272–279.

Stetler, C. B. (2010). Stetler Model. In J. Rycroft-Malone & T. Bucknall (Eds.), *Evidence-Based Practice Series. Models and frameworks for implementing evidence-based practice: Linking evidence to action.* Oxford: Wiley-Blackwell.

Titler, M. G. (2010). Translation science and context. *Research and Theory in Nursing Practice, 24*(1), 35–55.

Titler, M. G., Everett, L. Q. (2001). Translating research into practice: Considerations for critical care investigators. *Critical Care Nursing Clinics of North America*, *13*(4), 587–604.

U.S. Department of Health and Human Services. (2009). Code of Federal Regulations TITLE 45 PUBLIC WELFARE PART 46 PROTECTION OF HUMAN SUBJECTS. U.S. Department of Health and Human Services [Online]. Available at http://www.hhs.gov/ohrp/policy/ohrpregulations.pdf

U.S. Department of Health and Human Services. (2016a). Quality improvement activities FAQs. Available at http://www.hhs.gov/ohrp/regulations-and-policy/guidance/faq/Quality-Improvement-Activities/index.html

U.S. Department of Health and Human Services. (2016b). Human subject decision charts. Available at http://www.hhs.gov/ohrp/regulations-and-policy/decision-charts/index.html

White, K. M., Dudley-Brown, S., & Terhaar, M. (2016). *Translation of evidence into nursing and health care practice* (2nd ed.). New York: Springer Publishing.

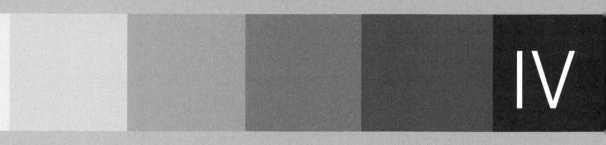

IV

Infrastructure

Creating a Supportive EBP Environment

Why be concerned about creating a supportive environment for evidence-based practice (EBP)? The most obvious answer is that new evidence is continually surfacing in nursing and medical environments. Practitioners must incorporate the tremendous increase in the generation of new knowledge into their daily routines for their practices to be evidence-based, yet there is a well-documented delay in implementing new knowledge into practice environments. The Agency for Healthcare Research and Quality (AHRQ) (Clancy & Cronin, 2005) cited 17 years as the average time from generation of new evidence to implementation of that evidence into practice. Additionally, for healthcare professionals to keep up with journals relevant to practice, every practitioner would need to read 17 articles per day, 365 days per year (Balas & Boren, 2000).

The dynamic and competitive U.S. healthcare environment requires healthcare practitioners who are accountable to provide efficient and effective care. This environment also mandates continuous improvement in care processes and outcomes. Healthcare, provided within the structure of a system or an organization, can either facilitate or inhibit the uptake of evidence. EBP requires the creation of an environment that fosters lifelong learning to increase the use of evidence in practice.

Because of the emphasis on quality and safety, many healthcare organizations have created strategic initiatives for EBP. Current national pay-for-performance initiatives, both voluntary and mandatory, provide reimbursement to hospitals and practitioners for implementing healthcare practices supported with evidence. Consumer pressure and increased patient expectations place an even greater emphasis on this need for true EBP. However, McGlynn et al. (2003), in an often-cited study, reported that Americans receive only about 50% of the healthcare recommended by evidence. Therefore, even with an increased emphasis on EBP, the majority of hospitals and practitioners are not implementing the available evidence and guidelines for care in their practices. This suggests an even greater imperative to build infrastructure that not only supports EBP but also infuses it into practice environments.

Three Institute of Medicine (IOM) reports have called for healthcare professionals to focus on EBP. In 2001, *Crossing the Quality Chasm: A New Health System for the 21st Century* called for the healthcare system to adopt six aims for improvement and ten principles for redesign: "The nation's healthcare delivery system has fallen far short in its ability to translate knowledge into practice and to apply new technology safely and appropriately" (p. 3). The report also recommended that healthcare decision-making be evidence-based, to ensure that patients receive care based on the best scientific evidence available and that this evidence is transparent to patients and their families to assist them in making informed decisions. The second report, *Health Professions Education: A Bridge to Quality* (2003), described five key competencies for health professionals: delivering patient-centered care, working as part of interprofessional teams, focusing on quality improvement, using information technology, and practicing evidence-based medicine. The third IOM report, *The Future of Nursing: Leading Change, Advancing Health* (2011), focused on the need to expand opportunities for nurses to collaborate with physicians and other healthcare team members to conduct research and to redesign and improve both practice environments and health systems to deliver quality healthcare. For this to happen, the report urges schools of nursing to ensure that nurses achieve competency in leadership, health policy, systems improvement, teamwork and collaboration, and research and EBP.

The American Nurses Association (ANA) revised *Nursing: Scope and Standards for Practice* in 2010, making a substantive change to the "Research" standard by renaming it "Evidence-Based Practice and Research." The new standard of professional performance requires that the "registered nurse integrates evidence and research findings into practice" (p. 51). The competencies are quite specific and hold registered nurses accountable to:

- Utilize current evidence-based nursing knowledge, including research findings, to guide practice
- Incorporate evidence when initiating changes in nursing practice
- Participate, as appropriate to education level and position, in the formulation of EBP through research
- Share personal or third-party research findings with colleagues and peers (ANA, 2010).

Other substantive changes throughout the standards emphasize the imperative for evidence in nursing practice and create a significantly stronger role for nurses to promote an EBP environment and advocate for resources to support research (ANA, 2010).

A new type of healthcare worker exists now—one educated to think critically and not to simply accept the status quo. Nurses from Generation Y, whose members are known as *millennials,* and Generation Z (http://www.socialmarketing. org) question current nursing practices, and "We've always done it that way" is no longer an acceptable response. They want evidence that what they are doing in the workplace is efficient and effective. These nurses are pushing the profession away from practice based on tradition and past practices that are unsupported by evidence. This push requires that evidence support all clinical, educational, and administrative decision-making.

This compelling need for EBP in the healthcare environment requires proper planning, development, and commitment. This chapter:

- Explains how to choose an EBP model for use in the organization

- Explores how to create and facilitate a supportive EBP environment

- Describes how to overcome common implementation barriers

- Discusses how to sustain the change

Choosing an EBP Model

It is critically important to establish a standardized approach to EBP inquiry in the organization. The establishment of a standardized approach, choosing a model, assures the team that appropriate methods have been used to search, critique, and synthesize evidence when considering a change in practice. Using a standardized approach is needed to implement best practices both clinically and administratively; identify and improve cost components of care; foster outcomes improvement; and ensure success of the EBP initiative.

Any EBP model or framework being reviewed for adoption should be carefully evaluated for the following:

- Fit and feasibility of the model with the vision, mission, philosophy, and values of the organization and the department of nursing

- Educational background, leadership, experience, and practice needs of the nursing staff

- Presence of any partnerships for the EBP initiative, such as a school of nursing or collaboration with other professions, such as medicine, pharmacy, and nutrition

- Culture and environment of the organization

- Availability and access to sources of evidence internal or external to the organization

The leadership team should appoint a group to champion the EBP process and review models using the characteristics in this list and other agreed-on criteria. Criteria for model review may include identifying strengths and weaknesses, evaluating assumptions, verifying ease of use, ensuring applicability for all clinical situations, reviewing examples of use and dissemination, and securing recommendations of other users.

Creating and Facilitating a Supportive EBP Environment

To move the EBP initiative forward, the organization's leadership must ensure that the appropriate infrastructure is available and supported. This organizational infrastructure consists of human and material resources and a receptive culture. Key assumptions regarding evidence-based nursing practice include these:

- Nursing is both a science and an applied profession.
- Knowledge is important to professional practice, and there are limits to knowledge that must be identified.
- Not all evidence is created equal, and there is a need to use the best available evidence.
- EBP contributes to improved outcomes (Newhouse, 2007).

Successful infusion of EBP throughout the organization must focus on three key strategies: *establish the culture, build capacity,* and *ensure sustainability*.

Establishing the Organizational Culture

Establishing a culture of practice based on evidence is a leadership-driven change that fundamentally challenges commonly held beliefs about the practice of nursing. This transformational change in culture typically occurs over a period of three to five years. During this time, EBP is embedded into the values, norms, and structure of the department of nursing and caregiving units through a planned and systematic approach.

Schein (2004) defines organizational culture as "patterns of shared basic assumptions that were learned by a group as it solved its problems of external adaption and internal integration, that has worked well enough…to be taught to new members as the correct way to perceive, think, and feel in relationship to these problems" (p. 17).

Thus, culture—a potent force operating below the surface—guides, constrains, and/or stabilizes the behavior of group members through shared group norms (Schein, 2004). Although organizations develop distinct cultures, subcultures also operate at the unit or team level and create a context for practice. Embedding a culture based on practice requires that nurse leaders at all levels explicitly challenge tradition, set expectations, model the use of evidence as the basis for decisions, and hold all levels of staff accountable for these behaviors.

The visible and tangible work of establishing a culture supportive of EBP requires revisiting the philosophy of nursing, developing a strategic plan, ensuring that leaders are committed, identifying and exploiting the use of mentors and informal leaders, and overcoming barriers.

Reviewing the Nursing Philosophy

A tangible way to signal a change to a culture of EBP and lay the foundation for leadership commitment is to review and revise the philosophy of the department of nursing. This statement should include three key points. The philosophy should do the following:

- Speak to the spirit of inquiry and the lifelong learning necessary for EBP

- Address a work environment that demands and supports the nurses' accountability for practice and decision-making

- Include the goal of improving patient care outcomes through evidence-based clinical and administrative decision-making

See Table 9.1 for an example of the philosophy statement from The Johns Hopkins Hospital (JHH) department of nursing. At JHH, the vice president of nursing and the directors wanted to ensure that the revisions in the philosophy resonated with and had meaning for the staff. After revising the document, they hosted an open forum with staff selected from all levels in the nursing department to provide input and feedback on the philosophy. This process highlighted the importance of this change, communicating leader commitment to EBP and to the part that staff would have in this change and transition.

Developing a Strategic Plan

Supportive and committed executive-level leadership, including the chief nurse executive (CNE), must be involved in the creation and development of an EBP environment. To operationalize the philosophy statement and build capacity for implementation of EBP, the organization's leaders must develop a strategic plan to identify goals and objectives, time frames, responsibilities, and an evaluation process. The plan also requires a commitment to allocate adequate resources to the EBP initiative, including people, time, money, education, and mentoring. As a strategic goal, EBP should be implemented at all levels of the organization. As the initiative rolls out, leaders need to check the pulse of the organization and be prepared to modify the strategy as necessary. To enable the process, they should identify potential barriers to implementation, have a plan to reduce or remove them, and support the project directors and change champions in every way possible. Figure 9.1 outlines the essential elements of a strategic plan for initial implementation of EBP. As EBP develops over time, the content of the strategic plan should reflect the maturation of the program.

The support and visibility of the CNE are paramount. The staff must see the CNE as a leader with a goal of infusing, building, and sustaining an EBP environment.

Table 9.1   Philosophy of The Johns Hopkins Hospital Department of Nursing

At The Johns Hopkins Hospital, we integrate the science of nursing, clinical knowledge, nursing judgment, and passionate commitment to quality care with the art of nursing, honoring patients' trust that they will be cared for with integrity and compassion.

In our practice...

> we are experts in the specialized treatment of illnesses;
>
> we pursue quality outcomes, advocating in the best interest of our patients;
>
> we embrace the responsibility of autonomous practice and commit to a collaborative approach to patient care;
>
> we seek, appraise, and incorporate the best evidence to support our practice;
>
> we master the application of healthcare technology;
>
> we pursue excellence, creativity, and innovation.

On behalf of patients and families...

> we pledge compassionate care throughout a patient's illness to recovery, discharge, or end of life;
>
> we use our skills to diagnose health concerns, intervene promptly, and monitor efficacy of treatment;
>
> we position ourselves as sentinels of safety and advocates for quality care;
>
> we honor individual uniqueness, embrace diversity, treat holistically.

As professionals...

> we bring intellectual rigor, ethical conduct, and emotional competence to our practice;
>
> we cultivate personal leadership and professional growth;
>
> we take the lead in our organization to improve patient care;
>
> we celebrate the talents of nurse colleagues, valuing positive relationships, shared governance, and mutual accountability;
>
> we advance our profession, locally, nationally, and internationally;
>
> we respect the diversity of persons, of disciplines, and of communities with whom we interact.

We treasure our heritage, celebrate our present, and engage the future.

We stand in the forefront of healthcare and nursing practice.

We stand for patients.

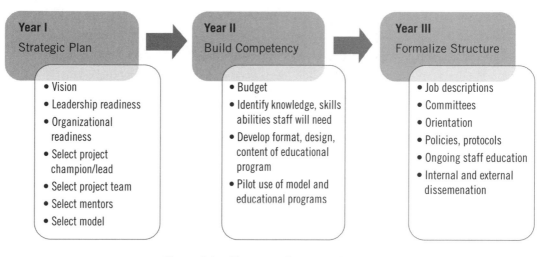

Figure 9.1   Elements of a strategic plan.

The organization's leadership can support EBP efforts best by modeling the practice and ensuring that all administrative decision-making is evidence-based. For example, if the organization's leaders ask middle managers for evidence (both organizational data and the best available research and nonresearch evidence) to support important decisions in their areas of responsibility, it is more likely that staff at all levels will also question and require evidence for their practice decisions. Additionally, all organizational and department of nursing clinical and administrative standards (policies, protocols, and procedures) need to be evidence-based and have source citations on the standards if a need to retrieve the reference arises. For example, at JHH, the infection control department implemented a policy regarding the use of artificial fingernails. Because nurse managers (NMs) were challenged with how to hold staff accountable for this change in policy, nursing leaders convened a group of NMs to conduct an EBP project on this topic. As a result, NMs were then armed with the best evidence on the risks associated with use of artificial nails and had direct experience with the EBP process and how it can strengthen administrative practice. With such leadership examples and activities, verbal and nonverbal EBP language becomes assimilated into everyday activities and establishes an evidence-based culture.

Finally, the CNE can further model support for EBP by participating in EBP change activities. For example, if the plan is to offer EBP education to the management group, the CNE can attend and introduce the session by discussing the organization's vision of EBP. The CNE's presence demonstrates the leadership's commitment to EBP and its value to the organization. Participating gives the CNE an appreciation for the process, including the time and resource commitment necessary for the organization to move toward an EBP.

Ensuring Committed Organizational Leadership

When leaders are actively involved and frequently consulted, the success of implementation, sustainability, and a stable infrastructure are more likely. When leaders are not engaged, the change-and-transition process is more reactive than proactive, and the infrastructure and sustainability over time is less certain. Greenhalgh, Robert, Macfarlane, Bate, & Kyriakidou (2004) describe three styles for managing change and adopting an innovation such as EBP:

- Leaders "let it happen" by communicating a passive style where, for example, small pockets of staff may self-organize to explore and create their own process for engaging in EBP.

- Leaders "help it happen" when a formal group such as advanced practice nurses, acting as change champions, have invested in and defined an approach to EBP and have to negotiate for support and resources to implement it. Still, the leader is being pulled into the process by change rather than leading it.

- The "make it happen" approach is intentional, systematic, planned, and fully engages all nurse leaders in the process to ensure adoption, spread, and sustainability.

Identifying and Developing Mentors and Informal Leaders

Mentors and change champions have an important role in assimilation of EBP into the organizational culture. They provide a safe and supportive environment for staff to move out of their comfort zone as they learn new skills and competencies. Informal leaders influence the staff at the unit or departmental level. The presence and influence of both roles is a key attribute for sustainability and building capacity within staff. Because EBP is a leadership-driven change, leaders should identify and involve both formal and informal leaders early and often in creating the change and transition strategies so that they can serve as advocates rather than opponents for the change and model its use in practice.

Leadership must identify and select nurse mentors with care, choosing them from across the organization—different roles, levels, and specialties. Consider who within the organization has the knowledge and skills to move an EBP initiative forward, can offer the best support, and has the most at stake to see that EBP is successful. Building the skills and knowledge of mentors should take into account such questions as, "How will the mentors be trained? Who will provide the initial training? How and by whom will they be supported after their training is complete?" As the activities to build an EBP environment increase, the leadership needs to diffuse education and mentoring activities throughout the nursing staff. The key to success is to increase buy-in by involving as many staff as possible to champion the EBP process by focusing on a problem that is important to them.

You can develop mentors in many ways. Initially, if the organization has not yet developed experts within their staff, it can find mentors through collaborative opportunities outside of the organization such as partnerships with schools of nursing or consultation with organizations and experts who have developed models. After internal expertise is established, the implementation of EBP throughout the organization results in a self-generating mechanism for developing mentors. For example, members of committees who participate in EBP projects guided by a mentor quickly become mentors to other staff, committees, or groups who are engaged in EBP work. EBP fellowships are another way to develop mentors where the fellow gains skills to lead and consult with staff groups within their home department or throughout the organization.

Evidence indicates that nurses, when facing a clinical concern, prefer asking a colleague rather than searching a journal, book, or the Internet for the answer. Colleagues sought out are often informal leaders, and evidence indicates that these informal leaders—opinion leaders and change champions—are effective in changing behaviors of teams if used in combination with education and performance feedback (Titler, 2008). Formal leaders differ from informal leaders in that formal leaders have position power, whereas informal leaders' power is derived from their status, expertise, and opinions within a group.

Opinion leaders are the go-to persons with a wide sphere of influence whom peers would send to represent them, and they are "viewed as a respected source of influence, considered by [peers] as technically competent, and trusted to judge the fit between the innovation [EBP] and the local [unit] situation. …[O]pinion leaders' use of the innovation [EBP] influences peers and alters group norms" (Titler, 2008, pp. 1–118). Change champions have a similar impact, but they differ in that, although they practice on the unit, they are not part of the unit staff. They circulate information, encourage peers to adopt the innovation, orient staff to innovations, and are persistent and passionate about the innovation (Titler, 2008).

The identification of champions can occur at two levels. The first is at the organizational level. At JHH, nursing leaders have successfully used clinical leadership roles such as clinical nurse specialists, wound care specialists, or safety nurse specialists as change champions. The second group of champions is at the departmental level and includes departmental nursing committee members who are expert clinicians whom the staff see as role models for professional practice and who can hold staff accountable. They are nurses committed to clinical inquiry and, many times, are initially identified because of their interest in the topic or issue for an EBP project or because they are skillful collaborators and team players.

The critical role of mentor and informal leaders in facilitating EBP and translating the evidence into practice has been the focus of significant work (Dearholt, White, Newhouse, Pugh, & Poe, 2008; Titler, 2008). The nursing literature supports that mentoring and facilitation are needed throughout the EBP process to help nurses be successful and to promote excellence (Block, Claffey, Korow, & McCaffrey, 2005; Carroll, 2004; Owens & Patton, 2003).

The Johns Hopkins Nursing Experience

After the JHNEBP Model was developed and ready for testing, the first group to receive education and training was the post-anesthesia care unit (PACU) staff. They were chosen for three reasons: The nurse manager was committed to EBP, the PACU had a well-established professional practice with expectations of staff nurse involvement in unit activities, and nurses had two hours of protected time scheduled each week, which could be used for the training. The PACU staff proposed to examine a priority administrative and clinical practice issue related to cost, volume, satisfaction, and throughput. The question generated by the staff was, "Should ambulatory adults void before being discharged from the PACU?"

The EBP process began with education classes held in short weekly or biweekly sessions. Each week, the PACU staff was asked to evaluate the education, the model, and their satisfaction with the process. They were asked the following questions:

- Is the model clear, usable, adequate, and feasible?
- Is the staff satisfied with the evidence-based process?
- Is the staff satisfied with the outcome of the process?

The results demonstrated significant differences across time in the nurses' perceptions of the adequacy of the EBP resources, the feasibility of the process, and their satisfaction with the process and outcome. Figure 9.2 describes the mean changes in evaluation responses across time. After the initial training, nurses began the process with positive perceptions; these dropped significantly in all three areas when they began to use the model to search and evaluate evidence independently. At the end of five education sessions, the nurses' perceptions of the adequacy of EBP resources, the feasibility of the process, and their satisfaction with the process and outcome returned to levels higher than their initial ratings.

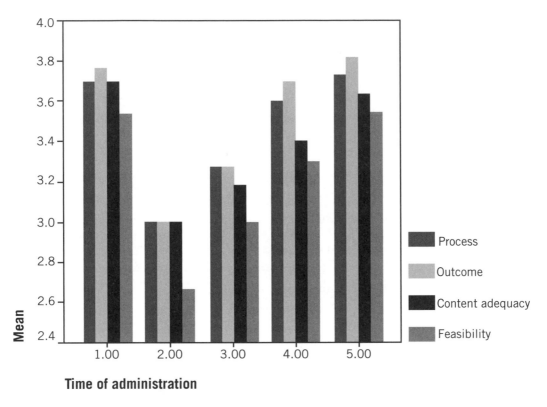

Figure 9.2   Nurse evaluation of pilot implementation of the JHNEBP Model.

These results support the need for mentorship during the EBP process as nurses learn new skills, including the research- and evidence-appraisal work (Newhouse, Dearholt, Poe, Pugh, & White, 2005). At the end of the pilot, the EBP leadership team concluded that staff nurses can effectively use the JHNEBP Model with the help of knowledgeable mentors and that implementation of a practical EBP model is necessary to translate research into practice. The evaluation also included qualitative responses that showed enthusiasm for the EBP process and a renewed sense of professionalism and accomplishment among the nurses. Indicators of success of an environment supportive of nursing inquiry included the following conditions:

- Staff has access to nursing reference books and the Internet on the patient care unit.

- Journals are available in hard copy or online.

- A medical and nursing library is available.

- Knowledgeable library personnel are available to support staff and assist with evidence searches.

- Other resources for inquiry and EBP are available.

Estabrooks (1998) surveyed staff nurses about their use of various sources of knowledge. She found that the sources used most often by nurses were their own experience, other workplace sources, physicians, intuition, and practices that have worked for years. Nurses ranked literature, texts, or journals in the bottom five of all sources accessed for information. Pravikoff, Tanner, and Pierce (2005) studied EBP readiness among nurses and found that 61% of nurses needed to look up clinical information at least once per week. However, 67% of nurses always or frequently sought information from a colleague instead of a reference text, and 83% rarely or never sought a librarian's assistance. If an organization provides resources for practice inquiry and creates an expectation of their use, EBP can flourish. Those who do not provide such resources must address this critical need.

Overcoming Barriers

One ongoing responsibility of leadership is to identify and develop a plan to overcome barriers to the implementation and maintenance of an EBP environment. This responsibility cannot be taken lightly and must be a part of the implementation plan.

Those involved in EBP have repeatedly cited *time constraints* as a barrier that prevents implementation of EBP and the continued use of an investigative model for practice. Providing clinical release time to staff participating in an EBP project is essential. Experience shows that staff need time to think about and discuss the EBP project, to read the latest evidence, and to appraise the level and quality of that evidence. Reading research and critiquing evidence is challenging and demanding work for most nurses and requires blocks of time set aside for effective work. It cannot be done in stolen moments away from the patients or in brief, 15-minute intervals. Nurses need uninterrupted time away from the clinical unit.

A *lack of supportive leadership* for EBP is another major barrier to the creation and maintenance of an EBP environment. Leadership can be facilitated through the vision, mission, philosophy, and strategic plan. The top leaders must incorporate EBP into their roles and normative behavior. To create a culture of organizational support for EBP, the day-to-day language must be consistent with using evidence and be a part of the organizational values. That is, leaders must *talk the talk*—making a point to ask, "Where is the evidence?" Leaders must also *walk the talk,* demonstrating daily a regard for evidence in their actions and behaviors. Does the organization value science and research and hold its staff accountable for using the best evidence in practice and clinical decision-making? Do leaders question whether routine decisions are made using the best possible data and evidence or using experience or history, financial restrictions, or even emotion? Do leaders themselves use the best evidence available for administrative decision-making? This can easily be seen if one looks at the titles of administrative staff within the organization. Does the organizational chart reflect a leader for departments such as research and quality improvement?" To whom do they report? Are these roles centralized or decentralized in the organizational structure?

A *lack of organizational infrastructure* to support EBP is another significant barrier. Resources, in terms of people, money, and time, need to be negotiated and allocated to support the initiative. Staff must be able to access library resources, computers, and current evidence in online database resources. Experts, such as the champions and mentors, must also be part of the available infrastructure.

Nurses themselves can be a significant barrier to implementing EBP. They often lack the skills, knowledge, and confidence to read results of research studies and translate them into practice. Some nurses also may resist EBP through negative attitudes and skepticism toward research. In some organizations, nurses may feel they have limited authority to make or change practice decisions and are skeptical that anything can result from the pursuit of evidence. Another potential barrier is the relationships of staff nurses with other nurses in the organizational hierarchy, such as clinical nurse specialists, and with physicians and other professional staff.

Barriers that come from nurses are best dealt with through prevention and planning to assess and identify staff needs. The EBP leaders, champions, and mentors can support the staff throughout the EBP process to incorporate the changes into practice. Professionals need to value each others' contribution to patient care and clinical decision-making. If the input of all staff, especially that of nurses, is not valued, a lack of interest and confidence in participating in an EBP initiative is the result.

Lack of communication is a common barrier to implementation of any change, but it is particularly detrimental to EBP initiatives. This barrier can be overcome by using the strategies in the design of a communication plan for an EBP initiative. As the staff develops EBP and approaches the clinical environment with critical thinking, they want to know that what they are doing is valued. The staff expects leaders to be responsive and open to their concerns or questions as the change is implemented. Staff will take ownership of the change if they sense that their leaders are partners in the change process.

A final barrier is *lack of incentives,* or rewards, in the organization for support of an EBP environment. Some think that staff should not have to be rewarded for doing their jobs. Leaders should consider, however, whether the organization's system includes incentives or disincentives and whether an accountability-based environment exists. Establishing an EBP environment and continuing EBP project work is challenging and requires a level of commitment on the part of all involved. Incentives can be dealt with in several areas already discussed: communication, education and mentoring, job descriptions, and evaluation tools. The leadership team should understand the need for such incentives and plan for recognition and rewards that are a part of the EBP implementation process. These are crucial discussion points during the planning, implementation, and maintenance of the change.

Leading Change and Managing Transition

A key factor for success when undergoing a culture change is that nurse leaders and those assigned to implement the change understand the difference between change and transition (see Table 9.2) and how to *lead* change and *manage* transitions (Bridges, 2016); this understanding provides insights on how to overcome the barriers discussed earlier.

Table 9.2   Definitions of Change and Transition

Change	An event that starts, stops, and occurs external to us
Transition	An emotional or psychological process that occurs internally—inside the hearts and minds of staff as they come to grips with the new way of doing things

Change is an event that has clear and tangible starting and stopping points. For example, a staff-led EBP project finds that patients and families prefer clinical staff to wear color-coded scrubwear to distinguish among team members. Based on this evidence, a decision is made to change to standard colors for scrubwear for all clinical staff. This is change—it begins with selecting colors for clinicians and ends when staff begin wearing the new scrubs. *Transition*, on the other hand, involves "letting go" of something familiar, valued, or treasured, which generates a feeling of loss. When staff are labeled "resistant to change," it is more accurately the transition they are resisting—the emotional process. Though change can take place in a short period, the time trajectory for transitions is different for each person and is defined by their emotional state at any given moment. So, to understand why some staff may resist change, leaders of the change have to understand what staff will have to let go of if a recommendation is made to standardize scrubwear.

The amount of planning for change and transition is directly related to the scope and complexity of the change and the amount of spread. Some changes may consist of simple, straightforward communication or educational "fast facts" on a device such as switching from use of a flutter valve to an incentive spirometer on a post-operative surgical unit. Or it may be complex, multifaceted, and hospital-wide, such as implementation of a nurse-managed heparin protocol that impacts nurse and physician responsibilities and workflow across the hospital. In either situation, knowing the difference between change and transition is important to success.

Strategies for Managing Transitions

Strategies for managing change are concrete and are guided by tactical plans such as those outlined in Appendix A. However, when change activities spark resistance, it is a clue that the staff are dealing with transition—the human side of the change. Resistance to change is how feelings of loss are manifested, and these are not always concrete. Losses may be related to attitudes, expectations, and assumptions—all of which make up staff comfort zones and provide them with a sense of routine and familiarity in what they do every day.

One way to head off resistance is to talk with staff about what they feel they stand to lose in doing things a new way—in other words, assess their losses. Another strategy to help staff move through the transition is to describe the change in as much detail as possible and to be specific so that staff can form a clear picture of where the transition will lead, why, and what part they play. In assessing loss, leaders need to think of individuals and groups that will be affected by the change both directly and downstream of the practice or process that is being changed. Because transitions are subjective experiences, not all staff will perceive and express the same losses. Examples of the range of losses include competence, routines, relationships, status, power, meaning to their work, turf, group membership, and personal identity (Bridges, 2016). Specific strategies to address these transitions include:

- Talk with staff openly to understand their perceptions of what is ending. Front-line clinicians have enormous wisdom, and what they see as problems with the change should be respected and tapped into by valuing rather than judging their dissent. Do this simply, directly, and with empathy. For example, say, "I see your hesitation in supporting the new scrubwear decision. Help me understand why." In the end, staff are likely to move through the transition more quickly if given the chance to talk openly about their losses.

- Because culture is local, tailor *how* the change is implemented to the context of the care-giving unit where staff work; staff need to own this action locally. This is one reason that informal leaders and change champions are important.

- Clarify what is staying the same, to minimize overgeneralization and overreaction to the change.

- After acknowledging the loss, honor the past for what has been accomplished. Present the change as a concept that builds on this past. One way to do this is with symbolic events or rituals that can be powerful markers of honoring the past. For example, staff may create a quilt or collage of pieces or patterns of their scrubwear or write on a large poster in the break room to mark what they are letting go.

- It is human nature for staff to complain, before they accept the new way of doing things. Avoid arguing about the statements you hear, because it shuts down communication; rather, liberally use your active listening skills. Understanding is more important than agreement. Be transparent, and let staff know when you don't know the answer; commit to finding out.

Do not underestimate the significance of communication in the change-and-transition process. Communication is essential in building broad support at both the organizational and the local levels. A key strategy is to be transparent and say everything more than once. Because of the amount of information that staff are exposed to, they need to hear it multiple times before they begin to pay attention. Bridges (2016) recommends a rule of thumb as six times, six different ways, focused at the local level in explicit terms. For staff to see the outcome of the change and move through the transition, follow these four communication guidelines:

1. Describe clearly where you are going with the change; if people understand what the *purpose* is, and the problem that led to the change, they will be better able to manage the uncertainty that comes with transition.

2. One outcome of communication is to leave staff with a clear, specific *picture* of what things will look like when the change is completed: What will the new workflow be? How will it look? What will it feel like? Who are the new players?

3. Explain the *plan* for change in as much detail as you have at the time; be transparent—if you don't know something, say so, and always follow with when, or what you will need, to answer their question at a later time.

4. People own what they create, so let staff know what you need from them, what *part* they will have, and where they will have choices or input.

Building Capacity

Building capacity refers to arming staff with the knowledge, skills, and resources to procure and judge the value of evidence and translate it into practice. Developing competency in using and applying EBP is best accomplished through education and direct practice gained through work on interprofessional teams.

Developing EBP Skills and Knowledge

The most popular format for EBP education programs at JHH is the one-day workshop. The morning session covers EBP concepts, the *JHNEBP Model and Guidelines*, and evidence searching and appraisal techniques. In the afternoon, attendees critique and appraise the evidence for an EBP question and decide, as a group, whether a practice change is warranted based on the evidence available to them. The one-day workshops have been implemented successfully in many settings outside of Johns Hopkins, including in rural, community, and nonteaching hospitals and other large academic medical centers. The educational topical outline for the one-day workshop is shown in Table 9.3.

Table 9.3   One-Day Workshop Topics and Objectives

Subject Area	Objectives
Introduction to EBP	Explain the origins of EBP Discuss the importance of EBP Define EBP
Guidelines for Implementation	Describe the JHNEBP Model Discuss plans for using the model Explain the steps in the process Discuss how to develop an answerable question
Appraising Evidence	Describe the different levels of evidence Determine where to look for evidence
Searching for Evidence	Discuss library services: How to have a search run by the library How to order articles How to do a basic literature search
Appraising the Evidence Application	Provide explanation of the evidence appraisal forms Facilitate group appraisal or evaluation of assigned articles Discuss appraisal of level and quality of each article Complete individual and overall evidence summary forms
Summarizing the Evidence and Beyond	Facilitate discussion of synthesis of the evidence Determine whether practice changes are indicated based on the evidence Describe fit, feasibility, and appropriateness of practice change Discuss how the practice change can be implemented Discuss how changes can be evaluated

Interprofessional Collaboration

In today's team-focused healthcare environment, interprofessional collaboration for the evaluation and dissemination of evidence in the healthcare work setting is a high priority because many practice changes involve not only nurses but also physicians, other allied health professionals, administrators, and policymakers. A conference held in February 2011 in Washington, DC—sponsored by the Health Resources and Services Administration (HRSA), Josiah Macy Jr. Foundation, Robert Wood Johnson Foundation, ABIM Foundation, and Interprofessional Education Collaborative (IPEC)—brought together more than 80 leaders from various health professions to review "Core Competencies for Interprofessional Collaborative Practice" (IPEC Expert Panel, 2011). The meeting's agenda focused on creating action strategies for the core competencies to transform health professional education and healthcare delivery in the United States. The fourth competency domain supported the need for interprofessional teams to provide evidence-based care: "Apply relationship-building values and the principles of team dynamics to perform effectively in different team roles to plan and deliver patient-/population-centered care that is safe, timely, efficient, effective, and equitable" (p. 25). When EBP teams are being developed, consider interprofessional participation and the identification and development of EBP mentors from the allied health professions.

Collaboration with a School of Nursing

It is widely recognized that education to develop skills and knowledge about EBP is essential for today's healthcare professional (IOM, 2003). This education is important at all levels of nursing education (AACN, 2006, 2008, 2011). The development of a collaboration with a school of nursing (SON) can benefit EBP for both organizations. The practice organization can provide real-life EBP questions for the students to use in their research courses. As a course assignment and using the questions provided by the collaborating SON, nursing students can search and critique the available evidence from PubMed and CINAHL to inform the practice question. The students can prepare a summary of the evidence, synthesize the findings, and make general recommendations for the practice organization to evaluate and consider translating to their practice.

EBP is an essential competency for Doctor of Nursing Practice (DNP) programs. Most DNP projects use the EBP process to evaluate the strength of evidence for translation into practice to solve a practice or administrative problem. PhD programs require that students understand the EBP process and use results to generate new knowledge for the profession. The collaboration between DNP and PhD graduates provides a strong team approach to improve clinical practice. Practice questions, issues, and concerns are often generated at the point of care by nursing staff, including DNP graduates. These practice questions result in evidence search, critique, and synthesis of findings. However, the synthesis of findings is not always strong or clear and requires further evaluation. This evaluation often involves a pilot study to generate new evidence. The involvement of the PhD-prepared research nurse is critical to the design of research and generation of new knowledge. This collaborative approach to practice between the profession's doctorally prepared nurses is the goal for practice organizations.

Finally, a collaboration with a SON can also foster the creation of faculty practice arrangements and faculty development. The development of a faculty practice can take many shapes, including both direct and indirect practice collaborations, depending on the needs of the practice organization and the SON. To more effectively integrate EBP concepts into the SON curricula and for professional development in the organization, a collaboration can be beneficial for both groups.

Sustaining the Change

At the beginning of an EBP strategic initiative, the organization's leaders must support and sustain a change in how the organization approaches its work. The leaders, mentors, and change champions and those responsible for the initiative must continually listen to the staff and be responsive to their comments, questions, and concerns. For EBP to become fully adopted and integrated into the organization, the perception that changing practice will improve quality of care and make a difference in patients' lives must be felt by all staff. The passion will be palpable when EBP becomes a part of the daily routine. Therefore, sustaining the change requires an infrastructure that aligns staff expectations and organizational structures with the strategic vision and plan for a culture based on evidence.

Setting Expectations for EBP

Setting role expectations for EBP through development of job descriptions, orientation programs and competencies, and performance evaluation tools is a first step in developing human capital for EBP and for hard-wiring the culture of practice based on evidence. These personnel tools should be developed or revised to emphasize the staff's responsibility and accountability for making administrative and practice decisions to improve patient care outcomes and processes. The tools must be consistent across the employment continuum. For example, the job description should state what is expected of the nurse in terms of standards and measurement of competence; the orientation should introduce the nurse to the organization and how standards are upheld and competencies are developed at the organization; and the performance evaluation tool should measure the nurse's level of performance on the standards with specific measures of competence. Table 9.4 provides examples of standards of performance and competence from the JHH department of nursing job descriptions.

Table 9.4   Excerpts from JHH Job Descriptions for Staff Nurses

CLINICAL PRACTICE

Nurse Clinician I: Applies a scientific basis or EBP approach to nursing practice

1. Complies with changes in clinical practice and standards

2. Participates in data collection when the opportunity is presented

3. Poses relevant clinical questions when evidence and practice differ

4. Consults appropriate experts when the basis for practice is questioned

5. Uses appropriate resources to answer EBP questions

6. Additional requirement for IM: reviews current evidence relevant to practice

continues

Table 9.4   Excerpts from JHH Job Descriptions for Staff Nurses   (continued)

CLINICAL PRACTICE

Nurse Clinician II: Applies a scientific basis or EBP approach to nursing practice

1. Seeks and/or articulates rationale and scientific basis for clinical practice or changes in standards

2. Supports research-based clinical practice (teaches, models, applies to own practices)

3. Participates in data collection when the opportunity is presented

4. Identifies differences in practice and best evidence

5. Generates clinical questions, searches evidence, and reviews evidence related to area of practice

6. Consults appropriate experts to answer EBP questions

7. Articulates evidence-based rationale for care

Nurse Clinician III: Interprets research and uses scientific inquiry to validate and/or change clinical practice

1. Evaluates research findings with potential implications for changing clinical practice, compares practice to findings, and takes appropriate action

2. Designs tools and/or participates in data collection and other specific assignments (e.g., literature review) in the conduct of research when the opportunity presents

3. Mentors staff to identify differences in practice and best evidence; generates clinical questions; searches evidence; and reviews and critiques evidence related to areas of clinical, administrative, or education practice

4. Serves as a resource and mentor in evidence-based discussions articulating rationale for practice

5. Participates in implementing EBP through modeling and support of practice changes

6. Incorporates EBP into daily patient care and leadership responsibilities

7. Participates in and supports EBP projects within the unit or department

RESOURCES

Uses critical thinking and scientific inquiry to systematically and continually improve care and business processes and to achieve financial goals.

Committee Structure

The committee structure is designed to promote excellence in patient care, education, and research by:

- Recruiting and retaining a diverse professional staff
- Establishing evidence-based standards of care and practice
- Promoting interprofessional quality improvement and research
- Advancing professional growth and development

These committees and their members took on the roles of EBP change champions and mentors for the department of nursing. Each committee serves a different but important role for implementing EBP throughout the organization.

Table 9.5 describes EBP functions for the department of nursing professional practice committees.

Table 9.5   Department of Nursing Committee Functions Related to EBP

Committee	Functions
EBP Steering Committee	Establishes strategic initiatives for EBP within and external to JHH and The Johns Hopkins University School of Nursing (JHUSON)
Clinical Quality Improvement Committee	Promotes evidence-based improvements in systems and processes of care to achieve safe, high-quality patient outcomes
Leadership Development Committee	Recommends and implements innovative evidence-based strategies for management and leadership practice
Research Committee	Supports discovery of new knowledge and translation into nursing practice

continues

Table 9.5   Department of Nursing Committee Functions Related to EBP (continued)

Committee	Functions
Standards of Care Committee	Promotes, develops, and maintains evidence-based standards of care
Standards of Practice Committee	Promotes, develops, and maintains evidence-based standards of professional practice

Communication Plan

A communication plan should be an integral part of both the EBP process and its sustainability. The plan should address:

- The goals of the communication
- Target audiences
- Available communication media
- Preferred frequency
- Important messages

Minimally, the goals for an EBP communication plan should focus on staff to increase awareness of the initiative, educate staff regarding their contribution, highlight and celebrate successes, and inform staff about EBP activities throughout the organization. Consider developing an EBP website within the organization's intranet. This website can be an excellent vehicle for communicating EBP information, including questions under consideration, projects in progress or completed, outcomes, and available EBP educational opportunities. The website can also serve as a snapshot and history of an organization's EBP activities and can be helpful when seeking or maintaining Magnet designation.

Finally, the communication plan can use online surveys to involve staff by asking opinions about potential or completed work, maintaining a finger on the pulse of initiatives, and developing EBP "messages." Messages can target the communication, link the initiative to the organization's mission, and give a consistent vision while providing new and varied information about the initiative.

After movement toward a supportive EBP environment begins, the biggest challenge is to keep the momentum going. To sustain the change, the staff must own the change and work to sustain it in a practice environment that values critical thinking and uses evidence for all administrative and clinical decision-making.

As resources are allocated to an EBP initiative, some may raise questions about expenditures and the costs related to EBP. To sustain the work of and value to the organization, EBP project work needs to be aligned to organizational priorities. It is helpful to identify EBP projects that improve safety or solve risk management problems; address wide variations in practice or in clinical practice that are different from the community standard; or solve high-risk, high-volume, or high-cost problems. Consider asking these questions: "Is there evidence to support the organization's current practice? Are these the best achievable outcomes? Is there a way to be more efficient or cost-effective?" Improvements or benefits to the organization could result in any of these important areas if EPB work identified best practices to improve outcomes of care, decrease costs, or decrease risks associated with the problem. Another way to show the cost effectiveness of EBP work is to improve patient and/or staff satisfaction or health-related quality of life. Sustaining the change also involves developing an evaluation plan to identify process and outcome performance measures that monitor implementation, commitment, and results. The measures should determine the usefulness, satisfaction, and success of the EBP environment. Are the initiatives changing or supporting current practice? What best practices or exemplars have resulted? Has the organization saved money or become more efficient? What performance data shows that this is making a difference to the organization? The evaluation plan should include a timeline and triggers that would signal when a modification of the plan is necessary.

Summary

We have learned many lessons in the development, implementation, and continual refinement of the *JHNEBP Model and Guidelines*. The need to create a supportive EBP environment is one of the most important lessons. Essential to that effort is recognition of the importance of capacity building for EBP. A supportive leadership is essential to establish a culture of EBP, including the expansion of infrastructure and the allocation of resources—such as time, money, and people—to sustain the change. Leaders set priorities, facilitate the process, and set expectations. The development of local mentors and champions contributes to the successful implementation of EBP and helps overcome barriers and resistance to EBP.

A culture of critical thinking and ongoing learning creates an environment in which evidence supports clinical and administrative decisions, ensuring the highest quality of care by using evidence to promote optimal outcomes, reduce inappropriate variation in care, and promote patient and staff satisfaction. Working in an EBP environment changes the way nurses think about and approach that work. As the nursing staff develop expertise in the EBP process, their professional growth and engagement begins a personal and organizational trajectory leading to evidence-based decisions, a higher level of critical review of evidence, and engagement in the interprofessional team as valued contributors.

References

American Association of Colleges of Nursing (AACN). (2006). *The essentials of doctoral education for advanced practice nursing*. Washington, DC; American Association of Colleges of Nursing. Retrieved from http://www.aacn.nche.edu/dnp/Essentials.pdf

American Association of Colleges of Nursing (AACN). (2008). *The essentials of baccalaureate education for professional nursing*. Washington, DC: American Association of Colleges of Nursing. Retrieved from http://www.aacn.nche.edu/education-resources/BaccEssentials08.pdf

American Association of Colleges of Nursing (AACN). (2011). *The essentials of master's education in nursing*. Washington, DC: American Association of Colleges of Nursing. Retrieved from http://www.aacn.nche.edu/education-resources/MastersEssentials11.pdf

American Nurses Association (ANA). (2010). *Nursing: scope and standards of nursing practice*. Washington, DC: American Nurses Publishing.

Balas, E., and Boren, S. A. (2000). Managing clinical knowledge for healthcare improvement. In J. Bemmel & A. T. McCray (Eds.), *Yearbook of Medical Informatics*, 65–70. Bethesda, MD: National Library of Medicine.

Block, L. M., Claffey, C., Korow, M. K., & McCaffrey, R. (2005). The value of mentorship within nursing organizations. *Nursing Forum, 40*(4), 134–140.

Bridges, W. (2016). *Managing transitions: Making the most of change* (4th ed.). Philadelphia: Da Capo Press.

Carroll, K. (2004). Mentoring: A human becoming perspective. *Nursing Science Quarterly, 17*(4), 318–322.

Clancy, C. M., & Cronin, K. (2005). Evidence-based decision making: Global evidence, local decisions. *Health Affairs, 24*(1), 151–162.

Dearholt, S. L., White, K. M., Newhouse, R., Pugh, L. C., & Poe, S. (2008). Educational strategies to develop evidence-based practice mentors. *Journal for Nurses in Staff Development, 24*(2), 53–59.

Estabrooks, C. (1998). Will evidence-based nursing practice make practice perfect? *Canadian Journal of Nursing Research, 30*(1), 15–36.

Greenhalgh, T., Robert, G., Macfarlane, F., Bate, P., & Kyriakidou, O. (2004). Diffusion of innovations in service organizations: systematic review and recommendations. *The Milbank Quarterly, 82*(4), 581–629.

Institute of Medicine (IOM). (2001). *Crossing the quality chasm: a new health system for the 21st century*. Washington, DC: The National Academies Press.

Institute of Medicine (IOM). (2003). *Health professions education: a bridge to quality*. Washington, DC: The National Academies Press.

Institute of Medicine (IOM). (2011). *The future of nursing: leading change, advancing health*. Washington, DC: The National Academies Press.

Interprofessional Education Collaborative (IPEC) Expert Panel. (2011). Core competencies for interprofessional collaborative practice: Report of an expert panel. Washington, D.C.: Interprofessional Education Collaborative.

McGlynn, E. A., Asch, S. M., Adams, J., Keesey, J., Hicks, J., DeCristofaro, A., & Kerr, E. A. (2003). The quality of health care delivered to adults in the United States. *New England Journal of Medicine, 348*(26), 2635–2645.

Newhouse, R. P. (2007). Creating infrastructure supportive of evidence-based nursing practice: leadership strategies. *Worldviews on Evidence-Based Nursing, 4*(1), 21–29.

Newhouse, R., Dearholt, S., Poe, S., Pugh, L. C., & White, K. M. (2005). Evidence-based practice: A practical approach to implementation. *Journal of Nursing Administration, 35*(1), 35–40.

Owens, J. K., & Patton, J. G. (2003). Take a chance on nursing mentorships. *Nursing Education Perspectives, 24*(4), 198–204.

Pravikoff, D. S., Tanner, A. B., & Pierce, S. T. (2005). Readiness of U.S. nurses for evidence-based practice. *American Journal of Nursing, 105*(9), 40–45.

Schein, E. H. (2004). *Organizational culture and leadership* (3rd ed.). San Francisco, CA: Jossey-Bass.

Titler, M. G. (2008). The evidence for evidence-based practice implementation. In R. G. Hughes (Ed.), *Patient Safety and Quality: An Evidence-Based Handbook for Nurses*. AHRQ Publication No. 08-0043. Rockville, MD: Agency for Healthcare Research and Quality.

V

Exemplars

Exemplars

The following section provides exemplars of how the Johns Hopkins Nursing Evidence-Based Practice (JHNEBP) Model has been used in practice. These exemplars describe the work of nurses to answer clinical questions, determine need for practice change, or guide policy development using evidence.

1

Establishing the Access in Minutes Team in the Adult Emergency Department

Madeleine Whalen, MSN/MPH, RN, CEN

Diana-Lyn Baptiste, DNP, RN

Barbara Maliszewski, MS, RN

The Johns Hopkins Hospital
Baltimore, MD, USA

Practice Question

Peripheral intravenous (PIV) access is one of the most common procedures performed in emergency departments (EDs) across the United States. Successful IV access is critical in providing timely diagnosis and treatments. Individuals with difficult venous access (DVA) may experience delays in care due to prolonged wait times for successful phlebotomy and IV access. In our adult ED, current practice dictates that a patient may receive two IV attempts from a nurse or clinical technician. If those attempts are unsuccessful, a more experienced staff member is allowed two additional attempts. If those are also unsuccessful, the patient's IV placement is escalated to an advanced practice provider. Though this strategy is in line with the Emergency Nursing Association (ENA) and Infusion Nursing Society (INS) standards, some patients experience significant delays in care—some waiting over eight hours for IV access or blood draws. The problem of DVA delays treatment and compromises patient comfort, safety, and satisfaction.

Given these threats to patient safety, a multidisciplinary team of clinical nurses, nursing leaders, clinical technicians, residents, attending physicians, and physician assistants convened to initiate an evidence-based practice (EBP) project to address the needs of patients with DVA. The foreground EBP question to be evaluated was this: Can the implementation of a dedicated difficult access team reduce the time from lab order to lab completion on patients with DVA as compared to our current practice in the adult ED?

Evidence

To gather evidence on DVA interventions, a literature search was conducted using the CINAHL, PubMed, and Google Scholar databases. A final selection of 22 articles was reviewed using the JHNEBP model. Two team members conducted independent reviews on all selected articles, which included grading and syntheses for all publications. Of the 22 articles, there were only two Level I studies, one randomized control trial, and one systematic review. Both studies provided high-quality (A) results to identify patients with DVA and promoted use of a dedicated team to decrease multiple attempts. A large number of articles were quasi-experimental studies, literature reviews, and expert opinion papers, graded at high (A) or good (B) quality. Eight Level II articles were quasi-experimental studies, some comparing standard practice versus use of dedicated difficult access teams to increase IV insertion success rates among adults in ED settings. Six of the eight quasi-experimental studies reported that using a dedicated expert IV team can significantly reduce the time to diagnosis and treatments. Level III (n=3), Level IV (n=6), and Level V (n=2) papers provided recommendations that included standards of practice, strategies for cost savings, and use of subject matter experts. The literature emphasized the importance of recognizing factors that contribute to DVA and supports the need for a designated difficult access team to reduce the number of attempts and avoid delays in treatment. Evidence synthesis revealed that:

- DVA is a condition among individuals who require two or more attempts for successful IV access:
    - 8–50% of children have DVA.
    - 14–35% of adults have DVA.
- DVA is associated with IV drug use, obesity, sickle cell patients, and chemotherapy patients.
- DVA negatively impacts patient safety and patient satisfaction.
- A dedicated IV team has been shown to decrease the necessity for advanced practice providers to place more invasive IV catheters.

- There are various approaches to determining expertise; self-nomination can be successful.

In reviewing the evidence for this project, there was a clear association between use of a dedicated IV team and a reduction in IV-site complications, a reduction in unsuccessful attempts, and an increase in timely placement and patient satisfaction.

Translation

Based on the evidence, the Access in Minutes (AiM) team was developed and put into practice in the adult ED. The team consists of self-nominated IV access subject matter experts who are available for consult Monday–Sunday 11:00 a.m.–3:00 a.m. when a patient's primary RN or clinical technician has had two unsuccessful IV placement attempts. Self-nominated subject matter experts received additional training on standards of practice and IV insertion techniques prior to implementation of this practice change. The AiM team is responsible for placing IV catheters and drawing blood, as well as for completing documentation to track multiple primary and secondary outcome measures. This practice change has been in place for six months and demonstrated a statistically significant reduction in lab order to lab completion time ($p < .001$). Additionally, the AiM team was able to reduce the number of IV attempts among patients with difficult access by 11%. These reductions mitigate the necessity for placing more invasive IV catheters, such as central lines, which often pose increased risks to patient safety and the costs to the institution.

Summary

The examination of evidence on interventions for patients with DVA proved to be a valuable experience for the EBP team. Through this process, we learned the importance of first identifying patients who have DVA and then initiating the appropriate team to promote successful IV insertion and venipunctures, with a goal of reducing number of attempts and decreasing time to treatment. These findings have been disseminated on the institutional, local, and state levels. Next steps include a research project to create a predictive scale to identify patients with difficult access to facilitate more timely activation of the AiM team.

2

Wipe Out CAUTI: Implementing Nonbasin Bathing to Reduce CAUTIs

Abigail C. Strouse, DNP, RN, ACNS-BC, NEA-BC, CBN
Director of clinical services surgery/neuro/ortho

WellSpan Health York Hospital, Department of Nursing
York, Pennsylvania, USA

Practice Question

Despite sustained efforts to implement best practices related to catheter-associated urinary tract infections (CAUTI) prevention, our hospital continued to see an increase in its CAUTI rate. After clinical review of each CAUTI event, it was apparent that more CAUTI events were associated with daily catheter care and maintenance than catheter insertion. Though CDC guidelines suggest that the use of antiseptics for catheter insertion is unnecessary, a specific method or cleansing agent for daily routine hygiene is not defined. Because most CAUTI prevention guidelines do not address catheter care and hygiene specifically, the best methods for bathing or cleansing adult catheterized patients to help prevent CAUTIs is unknown. As a result, a multidisciplinary CAUTI prevention workgroup began investigating innovative practices that focused on improving the daily care and maintenance of indwelling catheters, and quickly a study question arose: Do current bathing practices impact the transmission of healthcare–associated infections (HAIs) and CAUTIs among hospitalized adult patients? More specifically, could the use of plain disposable bathing wipes, instead of traditional basin bathing, reduce the incidence of CAUTIs for adult patients on a medical surgical nursing unit?

Evidence

The team performed a search of literature for articles published between 2000 and 2014 utilizing the CINAHL, Cochrane, OVID, PubMed, Virginia Henderson

Library, and Google Scholar databases. Literature pertaining to basin bathing, CHG (chlorhexidine) bath wipes, plain bath wipes, and associated outcomes were included. A title and abstract review eliminated a number of studies based on exclusion criteria, and the total number of studies included in the evidence review was 41.

Level of Evidence	Number of Articles	Quality A	Quality B
Level I	4	1	3
Level II	18	5	13
Level III	5	2	3
Level IV	0	0	0
Level V	14	1	13
Total	41		

The majority of studies and EBP projects included in the literature review were Level II and Level V and B-quality ratings, according to the JHNEBP Model.

The evidence indicated that bath basin bacterial contamination places patients who use basins at an increased risk for HAIs, including CAUTIs. Additionally, the removal of reusable bath basins can reduce patient exposure to harmful organisms, and the use of bathing alternatives, like CHG wipes and plain bath wipes, should be further investigated. Though the use of CHG and CHG wipes has been found to be effective in reducing central line associated bloodstream infections (CLABSIs) and surgical site infections (SSIs), no significant reduction in CAUTI rates when CHG wipes or CHG bathing protocols are implemented has been demonstrated. The evidence does support the use of plain wipe bathing to aid in the prevention of CAUTIs with little additional cost and high patient and staff satisfaction. For that reason, the removal of bath basins and the initiation of daily plain wipe bathing was the evidence-based intervention chosen for this EBP project.

Translation

Because the evidence supported the use of plain wipe bathing instead of CHG or basin bathing to aid in the prevention of CAUTIs, traditional daily basin bathing was replaced with daily disposable-wipe bathing on one 55-bed adult medical surgical nursing unit, and monthly CAUTI rates, medical supplies, and laundry costs were monitored over a 3-month period.

This relatively simple intervention posed no additional risk to patients or staff, and the target unit CAUTI rate decreased from 1.8/1000 catheter days during the pre-intervention period to zero following the implementation of disposable-wipe bathing. Decreased supply and linen utilization led to a savings of $0.16 per patient day, or a potential annual cost savings of $2,630 on the target unit. Findings were shared with nursing leadership and hospital administration, and in March 2016 the implementation of nonbasin bathing was adopted throughout the health system as the standard of care.

Summary

During the 3-month trial of disposable-wipe bathing, bathing times decreased, staff and patients reported satisfaction with the new bathing process, an overall cost savings was realized, and zero CAUTIs occurred. Though the transition from traditional bathing to wipe bathing was challenging for some staff to adjust to, its ease of use, associated cost savings, CAUTI reduction, time savings to nursing, and minimal risk supported the successful implementation of daily wipe bathing into practice. More importantly, a multidisciplinary team with limited knowledge of the EBP process had an opportunity to learn about EBP, assist in translating evidence into practice, and implement a practice change that led to improved clinical outcomes.

3

Drawing aPTT Samples from Central Lines While Heparin Is Concurrently Infusing

Daniel Hare, BSN, RN, PCCN

Margaret Witman, RN, PCCN

Candice Penaranda, BSN, RN

Jennifer Mayo, BSN, RN

Christina Ewing, BSN, RN

Barbara Palm, RN

Nicole Bahadursingh, RN

Ashley Ewald, RN

Capucine Dingle, RN

Heidi Mock, RN

Tania Fletcher, BSN, RN

Karen Keim, MSN, RN

Heidi Chroszielewski, MSN, RN-BC, PCCN

Mercy Medical Center
Baltimore, Maryland, USA

Practice Question

The practice of drawing an activated partial thromboplastin time (aPTT) from central lines while Heparin is concurrently infusing was inconsistent and not defined for frontline nurses. Nurse interviews validated the lack of clarity, including differences in the amount of time the Heparin was held prior to drawing the aPTT sample, the amount of normal saline used to flush the line prior to drawing the aPTT sample, and the amount of waste drawn prior to drawing the aPTT sample. A community search utilizing local Magnet hospitals revealed similar inconsistencies in nursing practice. An internal survey among clinical nurses was conducted, and the lack of procedural clarity had similar findings. To standardize practice, clinical nurses decided to implement an EBP process focusing on the procedural process of how aPTT samples are obtained from patients with central lines while Heparin is concurrently infusing.

A nursing team was formed to complete this EBP project to address the practice of drawing aPTT samples from central lines. The team included adult medicine nurses working on the progressive care unit, the unit educator, and the director of professional practice. The EBP question was this: In an adult hospitalized patient, what are the best-known practices for drawing blood from a central line to obtain an aPTT sample while Heparin is concurrently being infused?

Evidence

A literature search was conducted using PubMed, CINAHL, Cochrane, and JBI with the assistance of the medical librarian. Twenty-one articles were identified from the search, and 12 articles were appraised using the tools from the JHNEBP Model. There were 10 Level II articles and 2 Level IV articles. Overall, the findings showed that blood sample contamination influences aPPT results. Examples of techniques to prevent blood sample contamination may be flushing the line, providing a sufficient waiting period, and discarding enough blood before a sample is obtained. It was recommended to obtain aPTT samples from the peripheral venipuncture, if possible, and to use central lines with Heparin infusing as a last resort. Additionally, a step-by-step process based on evidence must be followed. Findings showed that the median aPTT difference when a specimen was obtained from a central line with a Heparin infusion port was –20.5 seconds (p=.008).

Translation

Based on the evidence, peripheral venipuncture is recommended as the first option, and CVAD with Heparin infusing should be used as the last resort. Because of the infrequent use of CVAD lines in obtaining specimens, practice needed to be changed by following the step-by-step process based on evidence to prevent blood contamination. A guideline was adopted to obtain aPTT samples from patients with central lines with a Heparin infusion. The new guideline was presented and approved by the practice and leadership councils.

Summary

Post-survey showed that nurses increased their knowledge and adherence to guidelines for obtaining aPTT samples from patients with central lines with Heparin infusing concurrently. As a team, the nurses were able to use the JH-NEBP Model to guide decision-making and development of a guideline for this infrequent procedure. The abstract has been presented formally within the organization with the focus on nursing process. Lastly, the use of the EBP process improved the nurses' attitudes toward evidence integration into practice, and the findings motivated the nurses to consider conducting research to measure patient outcome.

4

The Effectiveness of Sennosides to Decrease Constipation Post Uterine Artery Embolization

Dana Triplett, BSN, RN, CCRN
Deborah Phillips, RN, CRN
Suzanne Stiffler, BSN, RN, RN-BC
Jane Hauhn, RN, CCRN
Theresa Neskow-Logan, RN
Andrea Staiti, BSN, RN
Brad Cogan, MD
Robert Liddell, MD
David Sill, MD

Mercy Medical Center
Baltimore, Maryland, USA

Practice Question

In interventional radiology, all outpatients receive a follow-up phone call post-procedure from the interventional nurse coordinator. From these calls, an adverse trend was noticed with the population of patients who had undergone uterine artery embolizations (UAE) to treat uterine fibroids. These patients reported having difficulty with constipation that sometimes continued for five to ten days. Fibroids can press on the outside of the colon, impeding motility, and cause heavy menstruation requiring iron supplements. These factors alone put women at risk for chronic constipation. Additionally, opioids are commonly used to manage post-procedure cramping and discomfort; and patients often have limited mobility and minimal oral intake, which can further contribute to constipation. A retrospective data audit of 25 patients was done, and all 25 reported constipation with no bowel movements for six to ten days post-procedure. Unit staff discussed this trend at a unit shared governance meeting and agreed to initiate an

EBP project in search of a proactive treatment plan. The practice question posed was this: What are the best practices for decreasing the incidence of constipation post-UAE?

Evidence

As a part of the evidence search, the team surveyed six local hospitals. All six stated that their UAE patients reported issues with constipation post-procedure, but none of them had a pre-procedure protocol they followed to address this common complaint. A literature search was conducted by using CINAHL, PubMed, and JBI with assistance from the medical librarian. The search yielded 33 articles, and the team appraised and summarized 15 using the tools of the JHNEBP Model. After a more critical review, the group determined that only four of the articles were relevant to the EBP question. Although no articles dealt specifically with the topic of constipation in the uterine fibroid patient population, they did provide evidence to support and guide protocol development. The articles included one experimental study, two non-experimental studies, and one expert opinion study. All articles had an overall quality rating of high (A) or good (B) quality. All articles supported the claim that the combination of narcotics and surgery was a major contributor to constipation.

Translation

Synthesis of literature for translation of pre-procedure constipation treatment in pelvic surgery indicated that the laxative of choice for opioid-induced constipation was Senna-S. Based on summation of our literature search and collaboration with the interventional radiologists, a pre-procedure protocol was developed. Patients are assessed during procedural consultation for current bowel habits. Patients are then given instructions for the laxative protocol, ordered by the physician, to take two Senna-S tablets twice daily for the two days immediately prior to the UAE procedure. No laxatives are taken the day of the procedure due to NPO status. Patients are admitted for 24 hours following the UAE, and current admission orders include the use of Miralax or Colace.

Summary

Since implementing the new protocol, 14 patients have utilized this protocol for their UAE procedures. One of these patients was excluded from the protocol due to pre-existing bowel disease, and another patient was excluded because she preferred to use homeopathic remedies. Of the remaining 12 patients, 11 reported bowel movements within 72 hours (three days) post-procedure (91.7% percent) compared to five to ten days pre-protocol implementation. Only one patient reported a bowel movement six days post-procedure and reported that this was her normal bowel habit. An evaluation of the change in practice revealed that the patients who received the pre-operative bowel program benefited more by having shorter days of constipation.

The EBP project brought staff excitement and increased interest in the use of evidence. The team plans to continue to educate patients on the importance of following this protocol when preparing for a UAE procedure. The team has already started exploring the possibilities of taking this EBP project to the next level by conducting a research study to validate the effectiveness of the protocol.

5

Initiating Purposeful Hourly Rounding on an Inpatient Oncology Unit to Improve Patient Safety and Satisfaction

Laurie Bryant, MSN, RN, OCN, ACNS-BC
Irina Rifkind, MSN, RN
Sarah McCarthy, BSN, RN

**The Johns Hopkins Hospital
Baltimore, Maryland, USA**

Practice Question

Purposeful hourly rounding (PHR) is a patient-centered quality improvement initiative that uses five key interventions to improve patient satisfaction and to decrease fall rates and call bell use. Public reporting of patient satisfaction scores to improve quality of care is a national standard and is directly correlated with nurse responsiveness and patient safety. In addition, nurse satisfaction, work-flow, and efficiency can be hampered by patient call bell use. Hourly rounding literature suggests that purposeful hourly rounding can improve quality of care and patient and nurse satisfaction. Using the tools from the JHNEBP Model, the clinical nurse specialist was uniquely positioned to initiate an EBP project. The outcome measures were call bell rates, fall rates, and patient satisfaction with staff responsiveness.

The EBP question was this: How does hourly rounding affect patients' perception of nurse responsiveness, call bell usage, and fall rates?

Evidence

An evidence search was conducted by using PubMed and CINAHL. Twenty-seven articles were identified and reviewed. Of the 27 articles, no experimental studies were found—six quasi-experimental, six qualitative, one systematic review, and 12 expert opinion or quality improvement articles. Two were not applicable to the search. All the evidence appraised was given a high- or good-quality rating. The majority of the evidence reviewed focused on two outcomes: reducing patient use of call bells and increasing patient satisfaction. Fourteen studies measured call bell use. Eleven of those found a reduction in call bell use, and three found no change in call bell use.

Of the 17 articles on increasing patient satisfaction, 13 found an improvement in patient satisfaction scores, and four found no change. The evidence review suggests that additional studies measuring nurse satisfaction and patient pain levels are needed.

Translation

Using the literature as a guide, we planned to conduct rounds every hour from 0600 to 2200 and every two hours overnight using 5 Ps interventions. The literature used 4 Ps: Pain, Potty, Position, and Possessions. We added the fifth P, for pumps, because of the number of pump alarms on our inpatient oncology unit. Initially, we implemented a rounding checklist based on samples from the literature; however, we experienced low compliance and discovered existing technology that we could use to monitor hourly rounds. The clinical staff were educated about the benefits and implementation plan for hourly rounding at staff meetings. Upon admission to the oncology unit, patients and caregivers were informed about the rounding project using handouts and room signage that explained the 5 Ps: Pain is managed, Position is comfortable, Potty needs are met, Possessions are in reach, and Pumps (IV) are not beeping.

Summary

A high level of adherence with this practice change was achieved by monitoring the practice of purposeful hourly rounds, which included continued education of all staff and giving feedback about compliance; and also surveillance of call bell and fall rates and quarterly HCAHPS scores. Post-implementation call bell rates fell 40%, and fall rates decreased 44%. Patient satisfaction scores for staff responsiveness to toileting improved from 50% "always responsive" to 67%; and responsiveness to call bell, from 66% "always responsive" to 73%. Future goals include involving the patient in the PHR process and using an upgraded staff locator system and call bell technology to monitor compliance.

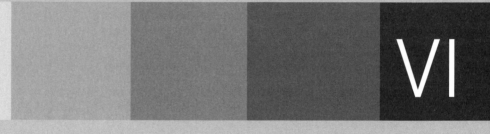

Using the JHNEBP Tools

Lessons from Practice: Using the JHNEBP Tools

EBP Project Example

This chapter provides several examples of how teams can complete the JHNEBP tools, and it gives helpful hints and guidelines to aid completion. The tools were completed using the exemplar "Wipe Out CAUTI: Implementing Non-Basin Bathing to Reduce CAUTIs," by A. Strouse (see Chapter 10).

Sample Tools

Appendix A: Practice Question, Evidence, and Translation (PET) and Project Management Guide

The EBP process begins with Appendix A (see Figure 11.1).
It provides a starting point and a concise overview of the steps in the process.

Initial EBP Question: Do current bathing practices impact the transmission of healthcare-associated infections (HAIs) and CAUTIs among hospitalized adult patients?

> Fill this in after completing Appendix B.

EBP Team Leader(s): Abigail Strouse

EBP Team Members: CAUTI prevention workgroup

Activities	Start Date	Days Required	End Date	Person Assigned	Milestone	Comment/ Resources Required
PRACTICE QUESTION:						
Step 1: Recruit interprofessional team	03/01/17	14 days	03/14/17	A. Strouse	Interdisciplinary team	Existing CAUTI workgroup
Step 2: Define the problem	03/15/17	7 days	03/22/17	Team	Problem	
Step 3: Develop and refine the EBP question	03/24/17	7 days	04/02/17	Team		
Step 4: Identify stakeholders	03/03/17	14 days	03/14/17	Team		
Step 5: Determine responsibility for project leadership	04/18/17	7 days	04/25/17	Team		
Step 6: Schedule team meetings	03/15/17	7 days	03/22/17	A. Strouse	Meetings arranged	Used existing CAUTI meeting time
EVIDENCE:						
Step 7: Conduct internal and external search for evidence	04/03/17	5 days	05/08/17	A. Strouse		
Step 8: Appraise the level and quality of each piece of evidence	05/09/17	21 days	05/30/17	Team		
Step 9: Summarize the individual experience	05/20/17	7 days	05/06/17	Team		
Step 10: Synthesize overall strength and quality of evidence	05/27/17	7 days	05/14/17	Team		
Step 11: Develop recommendations for change based on evidence synthesis: ▪ Strong, compelling evidence, consistent results ▪ Good evidence, consistent results ▪ Good evidence, conflicting results ▪ Insufficient or absent evidence	06/15/17	28 days	06/12/17			
TRANSLATION:						
Step 12: Determine fit, feasibility, and appropriateness of recommendation(s) for translation path	06/20/17	5 days	06/25/17	EBP Team		
Step 13: Create action plan	06/25/17	7 days	07/01/17	EBP Team		
Step 14: Secure support and resources to implement action plan	07/01/17	10 days	07/11/17	EBP Team	Approval	
Step 15: Implement action plan	07/01/17	7 days	03/14/17	EBP Team		
Step 16: Evaluate outcomes	07					
Step 17: Report outcomes to	08					

> Identify stakeholders early in the EBP process to secure their buy-in. Stakeholders are not generally members of the team, but receive ongoing communication about the progress of the project.

> Finding meeting times for the team can be a challenge. Look for opportunities to use meetings that are already scheduled (e.g., staff or committee meetings) to minimize the need for additional meetings.

> The project management tool is designed to be a roadmap that is updated throughout the project.

Figure 11.1   Completed Appendix A: Practice Question, Evidence, and Translation (PET) and Project Management Guide.

Appendix B: Question Development Tool

A successful EBP project depends on accurate problem identification and appropriate question selection. Teams should plan to spend substantial time completing Appendix B, and they may revisit it many times during the course of the project. Figure 11.2 shows segments of a completed Appendix B.

1. What is the problem?
Hospital continues to see an increase in CAUTI rates despite efforts to reduce rates; after-event reviews show more infections associated with catheter care than insertion; best methods for catheter maintenance are unknown.

2. Why is the problem important and relevant? What would happen if not addressed?
CAUTI is a preventable hospital acquired infection that brings patient t̶ addressed patient satisfaction will continue to decline and reimbursem̶

> It is important to clearly identify the problem you are trying to solve. Spending time looking at the issue from different angles and perspectives will help the team focus on the actual problem of interest. Often, teams start an EBP project with a solution in mind. Make sure your problem statement does not reflect solutions.

3. What is the current practice?
There are no standard practices on the unit for catheter care or bathin̶ each nurse's or technician's experience, many use basins for bathing.

4. How was the problem identified? *(Check all that apply.)*

✗ Safety and risk-management concerns	✗ Variations in practice compared to community standard
✗ Quality concerns (efficiency, effectiveness, timeliness, equity, patient-centeredness)	❑ Current practice that has not been validated
	❑ Financial concerns
✗ Unsatisfactory patient, staff, or organizational outcomes	
✗ Variations in practice within the setting	

5. What are the PICO components?
P – (Patient, population, or problem) Adult inpatients on Med/Surg units with indwelling urinary catheters
I – (Intervention) Identify standardized method for bathing and catheter care
C – (Comparison with other interventions, if foreground question) N/A
O – (Outcomes are qualitative and/or quantitative measures to determine the success of change) Decreased incidence of CAUTI among patients with indwelling catheters

> PICO format provides a useful structure for developing the EBP question. A background question usually does not include a comparison (C) because it seeks to find *all* best practices.

6. Initial EBP question ✗ **Background** ☐ **Foreground**

Do current bathing practices impact the transmission of (HAIs) and CAUTIs among hospitalized adult patients?

7. List possible search terms, databases to search, a

CAUTI, catheter, indwelling, infection, urinary, basin, bath

Acquired, care, clean

> Often, teams will begin the EBP process with a background question because it provides the team with all the best practices that may exist for a given problem. The search results for a background question are broad and provide a starting point when little is known about the topic.
>
> In this example, the team would look at all the ways to bathe patients or cleanse the area.

8. What evidence must be gathered?   *(Check all tha*

- ✗ Publications (e.g., EBSCOHost, PubMed, CINAHL, Embase)
- ✗ Standards (regulatory, professional, community)
- ✗ Guidelines

☐ Position statements

...inancial
...atient/

9. Revised EBP question

(Revisions in the EBP question may not be evident until after the initial literature review; the revision can be in the background question or a change from background to foreground question.)

Could the use of plain, disposable bathing wipes, instead of traditional basin bathing, reduce the incidence of CAUTIs for adult patients on a medical/surgical unit?

> The review of the evidence often leads to a foreground question, which is focused and specific, and compares two or more interventions. Here, the team is examining the use of cleansing wipes compared to basin bathing.

10. Outcome measurement plan

What will we measure? (Structure, process, outcome measure)	How will we measure it? (Metrics expressed as rate or percent)	How often will we measure it? (Frequency)	Where will we obtain the data?	Who will collect the data?	To whom will we report the data?
Rates of CAUTI	Incidence of CAUTI per 1000 catheter days	Monthly	Patient medical record	CAUTI team member	CAUTI team members and unit administration
Cost	Cost per patient day	Monthly	Unit budget	Finance	CAUTI team members and unit

> This outcome measurement plan was developed using the foreground question. Outcome measures selected in the PICO statement may change as the team reviews the evidence.

Figure 11.2   Completed Appendix B: Question Development Tool.

Appendix C: Stakeholder Analysis Tool

Teams should spend time identifying and engaging stakeholders early in the EBP process. Failure to adequately identify and engage stakeholders could negatively impact the project. Although stakeholders may change over the life of the EBP project, the team would be well served to perform a thorough assessment before beginning. Figure 11.3 demonstrates a stakeholder analysis (see Appendix C) for the sample project.

1. Identify the key stakeholders.		
✘ Manager or direct supervisor	❑ Professional organizations	✘ Administrators
❑ Finance department	❑ Committees	✘ Other units or
✘ Vendors	❑ Organizatio	
✘ Patients and/or families; Patient and Family Advisory Committee	✘ Interdiscipl (physicians respiratory therapists, or OT/ PT, for example)	

There are four roles that stakeholders can have. One stakeholder can have more than one role.

2. Stakeholder roles and responsibilities.

(The stakeholder roles—which include Responsibility, Consult, Approval, and Inform and their corresponding responsibilities, described here—guide completion of the table.)

Responsibility
- Carries out tasks to be completed
- Recommending authority

Consult
- Provides input (i.e., subject matter experts)
- No decision-making authority

Approval
- Signs off on recommendations
- May veto

Inform
- Notified of progress and changes
- No input on decisions

Project tasks	Stakeholder name	Stakeholder name	Stakeholder name
	Stakeholder role	Stakeholder role	Stakeholder role
Development of catheter care protocol	Cauti team		Frontline nurses
	Responsibility		Consult
Approval of practice change (protocol)		Clinical leaders	Managers/supervisors
		Approval	Inform
Catheter care education	CAUTI team	Nurses and technicians	Other units/departments

The team identifies individuals who have a vested interest, role, and responsibility in the project. For example, approval of the protocol falls to the clinical leaders, whereas the frontline nurses provide input and consult on content and feasibility of the protocol.

Figure 11.3   Completed Appendix C: Stakeholder Analysis Tool.

Appendix E: Research Evidence Appraisal Tool

When teams are appraising research evidence (Levels I, II, III), they use Appendix E: the Research Evidence Appraisal Tool. Hint: Use Appendix D (not presented in this chapter) for a quick overview for determining the level of evidence.

Figure 11.4 shows the appraisal of a Level I article using Appendix E.

		quality rating	_____IB_____
Article	In this section, the EBP team has indicated the Level of Evidence-I and the overall quality of this evidence-B.	ng protocol	Number: 3
Author(s): Jewett, R. and Martin, R.		Publication date: 2014	
Journal: American Journal of Nu	Numbering articles as you review them helps to keep the evidence organized. This is the third article the team reviewed. This number will also be used in Appendixes G and H.		
Setting: 2 participating centers: b academic medical centers		and size): 50 patients with randomized-25 to wipes and	
Does this evidence address my EE question?		Do not proceed with appraisal of this evidence.	

Is this study:

✗ QuaNtitative (collection, analysis, and reporting of numerical data)

Measurable data (how many; how much; or how often) used to formulate facts, uncover patterns in research, and generalize results from a larger sample population; provides observed effects of a program, problem, or condition, measured precisely, rather than through researcher interpretation of data. Common methods are surveys, face-to-face structured interviews, observations, and reviews of records or documents. Statistical tests are used in data analysis.

Go to **Section I: QuaNtitative**

❏ **QuaLitative** (collection, analysis, and reporting of narrative data)

Rich narrative documents are used for uncovering themes; describes a problem or condition from the point of view of those experiencing it. Common methods are focus groups, individual interviews (unstructured or semistructured), and participation/observations. Sample sizes are small and are determined when data saturation is achieved. Data saturation is reached when the researcher identifies that no new themes emerge and redundancy is occurring. Synthesis is used in data analysis. Often a starting point for studies when little research exists; may use results to design empirical studies. The researcher describes, analyzes, and interprets reports, descriptions, and observation

Go to **Section II: QuaLitative**

❏ Mixed methods (results reported in both numerically

Both quaNtitative and quaLitative methods are used combination, provides a better understanding of rese Sample sizes vary based on methods used. Data coll quaNtitative and quaLitative data in a single study or influence stages in the research process.

Referring to these descriptions, the team identifies the type of evidence before proceeding to the appraisal. Each type of research—quantitative, qualitative, mixed methods—has a separate section on the appraisal tool. In this example, the evidence is quantitative, so the team used Section I.

Section I: QuaNtitative

Level of Evidence (Study Design)

A. Is this a report of a single research study?		✗ Yes	☐ No Go to B.
1. Was there manipulation of an independent variable?		✗ Yes	☐ No
2. Was there a control group?		✗ Yes	☐ No
3. Were study participants randomly assigned to the intervention and control groups?		✗ Yes	☐ No
If Yes to questions 1, 2, and 3, this is a randomized controlled trial (RCT) or experimental study.	✗ LEVEL I		

⬆

Questions in this part guide the team in identifying the type of quantitative evidence. This study manipulated the independent variable, had a control group, and randomly assigned subjects. This is a randomaized controlled trial, Level I. The level of evidence is determined by the Yes and No answers provided under A.

If Yes to questions 1 and 2 and No to qu... question 1 and No to questions 2 and ... experimental (some degree of investig... manipulation of an independent varia... assignment to groups, and may have ...

| If No to questions 1, 2, and 3, this is nonexperimental (no manipulation of independent variable; can be descriptive, comparative, or correlational; often uses secondary data). | ☐ LEVEL III | | |

Study Findings That Help Answer the EBP Question

- Basin washing was shown to increase incidents of CAUTI
- Using clean wipes reduced CAUTI by 75%
- Patients showed a preference for cleansing wipes over basi...

Each appraisal section has an area for documenting the findings from a study or piece of evidence that is useful in answering the EBP question. These findings will later be transferred to Appendix G.

Complete the Appraisal of QuaNtitative Research Studies below, and assign a quality rating to your article.

Appraisal of QuaNtitative Research Studies

Does the researcher identify what is known and not known about the problem and how the study will address any gaps in knowledge?	✗ Yes	❏ No	
Was the purpose of the study clearly presented?			
Was the literature review current (most sources within the past five years or a seminal study)?			
Was sample size sufficient based on study design and rationale?			
If there is a control group:			
▪ Were the characteristics and/or demographics similar in both the control and intervention groups?	❏ Yes	❏ No	❏ N/A
▪ If multiple settings were used, were the settings similar?	❏ Yes	❏ No	❏ N/A
▪ Were all groups equally treated except for the intervention group(s)?	❏ Yes	❏ No	❏ N/A
Are data collection methods described clearly?	✗ Yes	❏ No	
Were the instruments reliable (Cronbach's α [alpha] > 0.70)?	✗ Yes	❏ No	❏ N/A
Was instrument validity discussed?	❏ Yes	✗ No	❏ N/A
If surveys or questionnaires were used, was the response rate $\geq 25\%$?	❏ Yes	❏ No	✗ N/A
Were the results presented clearly?	✗ Yes	❏ No	
If tables were presented, was the narrative consistent with the table content?	✗ Yes	❏ No	❏ N/A
Were study limitations identified and addressed?	❏ Yes	✗ No	
Were conclusions based on results?	✗ Yes	❏ No	

When assessing currency of the literature review, the team scans the dates of publications in the article references.

Go to Quality Rating for QuaNtitative Studies below

Appraisal of Systematic Review (With or Without Meta-Analysis)

Were the variables of interest clearly identified?	❏ Yes	❏ No
Were reports comprehensive, with reproducible search strategy?		
▪ Key search terms stated	❏ Yes	❏ No
▪ Multiple databases searched and identified	❏ Yes	❏ No
▪ Inclusion and exclusion criteria stated	❏ Yes	❏ No
Was there a flow diagram that included the number of studies eliminated at each level of review?	❏ Yes	❏ No
Were details of included studies presented (design, sample, methods, results, outcomes, strengths, and limitations?)	❏ Yes	❏ No
Were methods for appraising the strength of evidence (level and quality) described?	❏ Yes	❏ No
Were conclusions based on results?	❏ Yes	❏ No
▪ Results were interpreted.	❏ Yes	❏ No
▪ Conclusions flowed logically from the interpretation and systematic review question.	❏ Yes	❏ No

Did the systematic review include a section addressing limitations *and* how they were addressed?	❏ Yes	❏ No

Quality Rating for QuaNtitative Studies

Circle the appropriate quality rating below

A **High quality:** Consistent, generalizable results; sufficient sample size for the study design; adequate control; definitive conclusions; consistent recommendations based on comprehensive literature review that includes thorough reference to scientific evidence.

B **Good quality:** Reasonably consistent results; sufficient sample size for the study design; some control, and fairly definitive conclusions; reasonably consistent recommendations based on fairly comprehensive literature review that includes some reference to scientific evidence.

C **Low quality or major flaws:** Little evidence with inconsistent results; insufficient sample size for the study design; conclusions cannot be drawn.

Section II: QuaLitative

Level of Evidence (Study De

A. Is this a report of a single

Assessing the quality of the evidence is a subjective process based on a careful examination of the appraisal. There is no concrete number of Yes answers that lead to an A quality rating. Rather, it involves a process of using the appraisal results together with critical thinking and discussions among team members.

Evidence that is appraised as C quality is not used to make practice change decisions.

Study Findings That Help Answer the EBP Question

Complete the Appraisal of Single QuaLitative Research Study section below, and assign a quality rating to the article.

Figure 11.4   Completed Appendix E: Research Evidence Appraisal Tool.

Appendix F: Nonresearch Evidence Appraisal Tool

When teams are appraising nonresearch evidence (Levels IV, V), they use Appendix F, the Nonresearch Evidence Appraisal Tool (see Figure 11.5). Hint: Use Appendix D (not shown in this chapter) for a quick overview for determining the level of evidence.

Evidence level	Helpful hint: If the team seems to be answering No to many of the appraisal questions in either Appendix E or F, double-check that you are using the correct form or the correct section. For example, mistakenly identifying a quality improvement project (non-research) as a research study could lead the team to determine the evidence to be of poor quality when it was simply a matter of using the incorrect appraisal form.	
Article title: Catheter care in an inpa		
Author(s): Samuel, J., Gamma, B.		
Journal: Med/Surg Nursing, S516-S		
Setting: 2 participating centers: both academic medical centers		
Does this evidence address my EBP question?	✗ Yes	❏ No Do not proceed with appraisal of this evidence.

❏ **Clinical Practice Guidelines LEVEL IV**
   Systematically developed recommendations from nationally recognized experts based on research evidence or expert consensus panel

❏ **Consensus or Position Statement LEVEL IV**
   Systematically developed recommendations, based on research and nationally recognized expert opinion, that guide members of a professional organization in decision-making for an issue of concern.

■ Are the types of evidence included identified?	❏ Yes	❏ No
■ Were appropriate stakeholders involved in the development of recommendations?	❏ Yes	❏ No
■ Are groups to which recommendations apply and do not apply clearly stated?	❏ Yes	❏ No
■ Have potential biases been eliminated?	❏ Yes	❏ No
■ Does each recommendation have an identified level of evidence stated?	❏ Yes	❏ No
■ Are recommendations clear?	❏ Yes	❏ No
Complete the corresponding quality rating.		

❏ **Literature review LEVEL V**
Summary of selected published literature including reports of organizational experience and opinions of experts

❏ **Integrative review LEVEL V** ◀
Summary of research evidence and theoretical literature; analyzes, compares themes, notes gaps in the selected literature

■ Is subject matter to be reviewed clearly stated?	❏ Yes	❏ No
■ Is literature relevant and up-to-date (most sources are within the past five years or classic)?		
■ Of the literature reviewed, is there a meaningful analysis of the conclusions across the articles included in the review?		
■ Are gaps in the literature identified?	❏ Yes	❏ No
■ Are recommendations made for future practice or study?		

Sometimes, integrative reviews may be titled or referred to as systematic reviews. However, closer examination reveals they combine research evidence and theoretical literature.

Complete the corresponding quality rating.

❏ **Expert opinion LEVEL V** ◀
Opinion of one or more individuals based on clinical expertise

Expert opinion can come from one or more individuals, but does not include a consensus with a consensus statement developed by a group of experts or members of a professional organization.

■ Has the individual published or presented on the topic?	❏ Yes	❏ No.
■ Is the author's opinion based on scientific evidence?	❏ Yes	❏ No
■ Is the author's opinion clearly stated?	❏ Yes	❏ No
■ Are potential biases acknowledged?	❏ Yes	❏ No

Complete the corresponding quality

Teams often wonder how to differentiate between expert opinion and clinician experience. A quick Internet search may tell you if the person has previously published or presented on the topic. If you are unable to find anything linking them to the topic, you may consider it clinician experience.

Quality Rating for Organizational Experience (Level V)

A. **High quality**
Clear aims and objectives; consistent results ̶a̶n̶d̶ formal quality improvement or financial
evaluation methods used; definitive conclusion̶s̶ ̶a̶n̶d̶ consistent recommendations with reference to
scientific evidence.

> Notice there are different quality guides for
> the various types of nonresearch evidence.
> Choosing an incorrect rating guide may lead
> the team to mislabel the quality of a piece of
> evidence.

B. **Good quality**
Clear aims and objectives; formal quality improvement or financial evaluation methods used; consistent
results in a single setting; reasonably consistent recommendations with some reference to scientific evidence.

C. **Low quality or major flaws**
Unclear or missing aims and objectives; inconsistent results; poorly defined quality; improvement/financial
analysis method; recommendations cannot be made.

**Quality Rating for Case Report, Integrative Review, Literature Review, Expert Opinion, Community
Standard, Clinician Experience, Consumer Preference (Level V)**

A. **High quality**
Expertise is clearly evident, draws definitive conclusions, and provides scientific rationale; thought leader in
the field.

B. **Good quality**
Expertise appears to be credible, draws fairly definitive conclusions, and provides logical argument for
opinions.

C. **Low quality or major flaws**
Expertise is not discernable or is dubious; conclusions cannot be drawn.

Figure 11.5   Completed Appendix F: Nonresearch Evidence Appraisal Tool.

Appendix G: Individual Evidence Summary Form

As the EBP team completes the appraisal of evidence, each article or piece of evidence should be entered into Appendix G. This becomes the team's reference and synopsis of the evidence reviewed. Remember that each piece of evidence should be appraised by more than one member of the team, and together they reach a consensus on level and quality. Some groups may decide to enter each article as it is read and discussed, whereas others may wait until all articles have been appraised. Either way is acceptable. Figure 11.6 provides a snapshot of Appendix G and shows only a few of the articles reviewed. Note that evidence rated C-quality should not be used or transferred to Appendix G. The team should not rely on low-quality evidence to make decisions.

EBP Question: Could the use of plain, disposable bathing wipes, instead of traditional basin bathing, reduce the incidence of CAUTIs for adult patients on a medical surgical nursing unit?

Date: 2017

> Appendixes E & F direct you to number each piece of evidence. This is where that number is used.

> Findings that help answer your EBP question are entered here, directly from the appraisal tool.

> Enter the metrics identified from each source of evidence. These provide ideas for metrics the EBP team may consider to determine if the practice change was successful.

> Limitations include not only those identified by the authors, but also limitations the EBP team identifies. For example, if your population of interest is pediatrics and this article addresses adults, that would be a limitation to acknowledge.

Article #	Author and Date	Evidence Type	Size, Setting	Findings That Help Answer the EBP Question	Observable Measures	Limitations	Evidence Level, Quality
3	Jewett, R. & Martin, R. (2014)	RCT	50 patients were randomized 25 received basin and 25 received wipe	Basin washing was shown to increase incidences of CAUTI Using clean wipes reduced CAUTI by 75% Patients showed a preference for cleansing wipes over basin water	Incidence of CAUTI/1000 catheter days	Academic medical center with higher staffing levels	Level I Quality B
4	Samuel, J., Gamma, M., & Bean, B. (2013)		✗ N/A	Use of cleansing wipes should be univerally adopted Much preferred over basin cleaning by both patients and staff All staff should be trained in CAUTI prevention techniques		Limited evidence use pra dec	Level IV Quality B
5	Jackson, J. & Lyn, R. (2015)	Quasi experimental			Incidence of CAUTI/1000 catheter days	Ins Sar	
6	Finch, E. L. (2016)	Qualitative				Sm	
7	Woodrow, A. (2017)	Expert opinion	✗ N/A	Benefits of cleansing wipe			

Figure 11.6   Completed Appendix G: Individual Evidence Summary Tool.

Appendix H: Synthesis Process and Recommendations Tool

Once Appendix G is completed, the team moves into evidence synthesis. The synthesis process is described in Appendix H. Using this tool, the team outlines the overall quality of the evidence to answer the EBP question, including the number of sources for each level. This appendix is also where the team, through reasoning, evaluates evidence for consistency across findings; evaluates the meaning and relevance of the findings; and merges findings that may either enhance the team's knowledge or generate new insights, perspectives, and understandings. In Appendix H, the team identifies the recommendations for practice change. See Figure 11.7 for a completed Appendix H.

EBP [The total number of sources for each level is entered here.] reduce the incidence of CAUTIs for adult patients on a medical/surgical unit.

Ca...	Total Number of Sources/ Level	Overall Quality Rating	Synthesis of Findings / Evidence That Answers the EBP Question
Level I ■ Experimental study ■ Randomized controlled trial (RCT) ■ Systematic review of RCTs with or without meta-analysis	4	B	There was no significant difference in rates of CAUTI between basin cleaning and no care (2) Cleansing wipes had statistically significant impact on rates (3) Secondary analysis found a significant difference in the number of CAUTI cases in units where wipes are available (12)
Level II ■ Quasi-experimental studies ■ Systematic review of a combination of RCTs and quasi-experimental studies, or quasi-experimental studies only, with or without meta-analysis	18	A-B	In hospitalized adults, self-care for catheter cleansing is recommended (5) Notice the overall quality rating. It is not necessary to settle on one letter if the team concludes the group of evidence is between two grades. As you can see here, Levels II, III, and V have a mix of A and B quality overall.
Level III ■ Non-experimental study ■ Systematic review of a combination of RCTs, quasi-experimental and nonexperimental studies, or non-experimental studies only, with or without meta-analysis ■ QuaLitative study or meta-synthesis	5	A-B	Basin cleansing had significantly more infections (17) Cleansing wipes more cost effective (8,10)

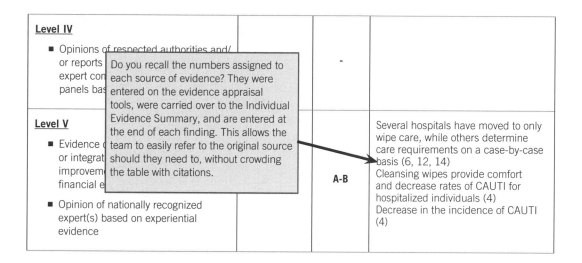

Level IV		-	
■ Opinions of respected authorities and/ or reports expert con panels bas			
Level V ■ Evidence or integrat improvem financial e ■ Opinion of nationally recognized expert(s) based on experiential evidence		A-B	Several hospitals have moved to only wipe care, while others determine care requirements on a case-by-case basis (6, 12, 14) Cleansing wipes provide comfort and decrease rates of CAUTI for hospitalized individuals (4) Decrease in the incidence of CAUTI (4)

> Do you recall the numbers assigned to each source of evidence? They were entered on the evidence appraisal tools, were carried over to the Individual Evidence Summary, and are entered at the end of each finding. This allows the team to easily refer to the original source should they need to, without crowding the table with citations.

EBP Question: Could the use of plain, disposable bathing wipes, instead of traditional basin bathing, reduce the incidence of CAUTIs for adult patients on a medical/surgical unit?

Based on your synthesis, which of the following four pathways to translation represents the overall strength of the evidence?

❑ Strong, compelling evidence, consistent results: Solid indication for a practice change is indicated.

✘ Good and consistent evidence: Consider pilot of change or further investigation.

❑ Good but conflicting evidence: No indication for practice change; consider further investigation for new evidence or develop a research study.

❑ Little or no evidence: No indication for practice change; consi develop a research study or discontinue project.

If you selected either the first option or the second option, continue.

> After determining they had good and consistent evidence, the team developed recommendations. These flowed directly from the synthesis of evidence above.

Recommendations based on evidence synthesis and selected translation pathway

Pilot the use of plain cleansing wipes on one med/surg unit

Remove basins from storage on pilot unit

Initiate daily plain wipe cleansing

Monitor for effectiveness

Are the recommendations:

✗ Compatible with the unit/departmental/organizational cultural values or norms?

✗ Consistent with unit/departmental/organizational assumptions, structures, attitudes, beliefs, and/or practices?

✗ Consistent with the unit/departmental/organizational

> Answering questions about fit and feasibility allows the team to determine the likelihood of success of the implementation. Not meeting all of the criteria does not mean the practice change cannot happen. However, it does indicate the need for further assessment and evaluation. For example, not having support available may mean you need to engage more stakeholders. Of course, recommendations that are not a good fit and/or feasible should not be implemented.

✗ Can we do what they did in our work environment?

✗ Are the following supports available?

  ■ Resources
  ■ Funding
  ■ Approval from administration and clinical leaders
  ■ Stakeholder support

✗ Is it likely that the recommendations can be implemented within the unit/department/organization?

Figure 11.7   Completed Appendix H: Synthesis Process and Recommendations Tool.

Appendix I: Action Planning Tool

Translating EBP findings into practice is multifaceted and is the fundamental part of the PET process—the reason why EBP projects are undertaken. Once the team has determined the fit and feasibility of the change, the next step is to plan for implementation. Appendix I provides an opportunity to identify strengths in the internal environment, potential barriers, and plans for mitigation. In addition, it prompts the team to confirm the available resources and funding prior to rollout. Finally, Appendix I guides the team to group the action planning tasks into critical milestones. Figure 11.8 shows the completed Appendix I based on the exemplar.

1. Complete the following activities to ensure successful translation:

✘ Secure a project leader.

✘ Consider whether translation activities require different or additional members. ←

✘ Identify critical milestones and related tasks.

✘ Identify change champions.

✘ Schedule time to complete

> Often, translation requires different team members than those who worked on the EBP project. It is not uncommon for members to be added at this stage.

able pre- or post-

2. Identify barriers to the success of the change, and then identify strengths that can be leveraged to overcome barriers.

Barriers	Resources or Strengths	Plan to Overcome Barriers by Leveraging Strengths as Appropriate
Need approval for implementing project in single med/surg unit as a pilot	Team members from CAUTI workgroup and pilot unit know the approval process for their department and different disciplines	Team members who know the process will submit protocol for approval
Education of large number nurses and technicians	Nurse educators and nurse leaders on pilot unit	Allow educators time to develop an education plan and implement
Equipment available	Supply coordinator for each unit	Supply coordinator to ensure adequate supply of wipes and remove basins

3. Consider whether or how this change will affect the following:

✘ Electronic health record   ❑ Workflow   ❑ Policies and/or procedures

4. Confirm support and/or availability of funds to cover expenses. (Check all that apply.)

❑ Personnel costs

✘ Supplies/equipment

❑ Technology

✘ Photocopying

✘ E...

❑ C...

✘ D...

❑ O...

> Identifying potential barriers and resources prior to implementation allows the team to take a proactive approach and take time to develop plans to overcome those barriers. It is helpful to match a resource or strength with every barrier (of course, you can have more than one strength for each barrier, too).

Figure 11.8   Completed Appendix I: Action Planning Tool.

Appendix J: Dissemination Tool

The final step in any EBP project is dissemination. It is important to communicate practice changes and results of EBP projects both internally and externally. Appendix J assists groups to craft messages suitable for each intended audience. Figure 11.9 provides an example.

1. Think about the project findings and practice change initiative. What is the most important information you need to convey?
Cleansing wipes are best practice over basin bathing. With implementation of change: ■ Over three months, bathing times decreased and staff and patients reported satisfaction with new process ■ CAUTI rate decreased from 1.8/1000 catheter days to 0/1000 catheter days. ■ The unit saved $0.16 per patient day (potential of $2630 per year)

2. Align key messages with audiences.

Audience	Key Message	Communication Method (see below)
Interdisciplinary stakeholders	Cleansing wipe use is best practice and has proven results	Internal meetings/in-services
Organizational leadership	Improved care and cost effectiveness stem from wipe use	Internal meetings/in-services
Departmental leadership	It is important to align the key message with the audience. People are interested in what the change means for them and how they may be affected. Carefully tailoring the content and message to the audience will ensure that these concerns are met.	
Frontline staff	Findings of EBP and rationale for changing way of providing catheter care; instructions for using wipes	Internal meetings/in-services
External community (publications, posters, and presentations)	Implementing best evidence resulted in a decrease in CAUTI rates and lower cost	Written publication External conference/podium presentation

3. Review examples below to identify appropriate communication methods.

Figure 11.9   Completed Appendix J: Dissemination Tool.

The tools provided in the JHNEBP Model provide structure and guidance to teams completing evidence-based practice projects. The tools are intended to walk the team through each step of the process and are meant to be completed in sequence. However, teams may sometimes need to step back and return to previously completed tools. For example, after an intial review of the evidence, the team may decide to change the EBP question from background to foreground, requiring a return to Appendix B.

VII

Appendixes

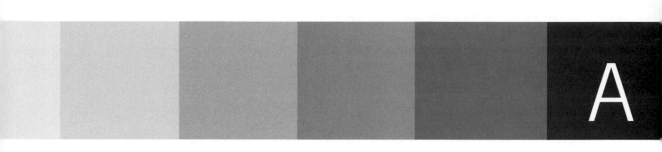

Practice Question, Evidence, and Translation (PET) and Project Management Guide

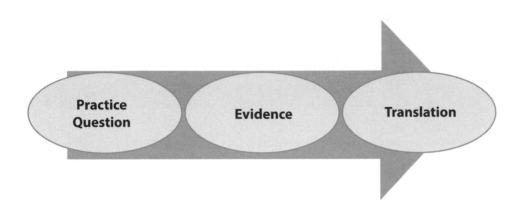

PRACTICE QUESTION

Step 1: Recruit interprofessional team.

Step 2: Define the problem.

Step 3: Develop and refine the EBP question.

Step 4: Identify stakeholders.

Step 5: Determine responsibility for project leadership.

Step 6: Schedule team meetings.

EVIDENCE

Step 7: Conduct internal and external search for evidence.

Step 8: Appraise the level and quality of each piece of evidence.

Step 9: Summarize the individual evidence.

Step 10: Synthesize overall strength and quality of evidence.

Step 11: Develop recommendations for change based on evidence synthesis.

- Strong, compelling evidence, consistent results.
- Good evidence, consistent results.
- Good evidence, conflicting results.
- Insufficient or absent evidence.

TRANSLATION

Step 12: Determine fit, feasibility, and appropriateness of recommendation(s) for translation path.

Step 13: Create action plan.

Step 14: Secure support and resources to implement action plan.

Step 15: Implement action plan.

Step 16: Evaluate outcomes.

Step 17: Report outcomes to stakeholders.

Step 18: Identify next steps.

Step 19: Disseminate findings.

Activities	Start Date	Days Required	End Date	Person Assigned	Milestone	Comment/ Resources Required
Initial EBP Question:						
EBP Team Leader(s):						
EBP Team Members:						
PRACTICE QUESTION:						
Step 1: Recruit interprofessional team						
Step 2: Define the problem						
Step 3: Develop and refine the EBP question						
Step 4: Identify stakeholders						
Step 5: Determine responsibility for project leadership						
Step 6: Schedule team meetings						
EVIDENCE:						
Step 7: Conduct internal and external search for evidence						
Step 8: Appraise the level and quality of each piece of evidence						
Step 9: Summarize the individual evidence						
Step 10: Synthesize overall strength and quality of evidence						
Step 11: Develop recommendations for change based on evidence synthesis: <ul><li>Strong, compelling evidence, consistent results</li><li>Good evidence, consistent results</li><li>Good evidence, conflicting results</li><li>Insufficient or absent evidence</li></ul>						
TRANSLATION:						
Step 12: Determine fit, feasibility, and appropriateness of recommendation(s) for translation path						
Step 13: Create action plan						
Step 14: Secure support and resources to implement action plan						
Step 15: Implement action plan						
Step 16: Evaluate outcomes						
Step 17: Report outcomes to stakeholders						
Step 18: Identify next steps.						
Step 19: Disseminate findings.						

Question Development Tool

1. What is the problem?

2. Why is the problem important and relevant? What would happen if it were not addressed?

3. What is the current practice?

4. How was the problem identified? *(Check all that apply.)*

- ❏ Safety and risk-management concerns
- ❏ Quality concerns (efficiency, effectiveness, timeliness, equity, patient-centeredness)
- ❏ Unsatisfactory patient, staff, or organizational outcomes
- ❏ Variations in practice within the setting
- ❏ Variations in practice compared to community standard
- ❏ Current practice that has not been validated
- ❏ Financial concerns

5. What are the PICO components?

P – (Patient, population, or problem)

I – (Intervention)

C – (Comparison with other interventions, if foreground question)

O – (Outcomes are qualitative or quantitative measures to determine the success of change)

6. Initial EBP question ❏ Background ❏ Foreground

7. List possible search terms, databases to search, and search strategies.

8. What evidence must be gathered? *(Check all that apply.)*

❑ Publications (e.g., EBSCOHost, PubMed, CINAHL, Embase)

❑ Standards (regulatory, professional, community)

❑ Guidelines

❑ Organizational data (e.g., QI, financial data, local clinical expertise, patient/family preferences)

❑ Position statements

9. Revised EBP question

(Revisions in the EBP question may not be evident until after the initial evidence review; the revision can be in the background question or a change from the background to a foreground question.)

10. Outcome measurement plan

What will we measure? (Structure, process, outcome measures)	How will we measure it? (Metrics expressed as rate or percent)	How often will we measure it? (Frequency)	Where will we obtain the data?	Who will collect the data?	To whom will we report the data?

Directions for Use of the Question Development Tool

Purpose

This form is used to develop an answerable EBP question and to guide the team in the evidence search process. The question, search terms, search strategy, and sources of evidence can be revised as the EBP team refines the EBP question.

What is the problem, and why is it important?

Indicate why the project was undertaken. What led the team to seek evidence? Ensure that the problem statement defines the actual problem and does not include a solution. Whenever possible, quantify the extent of the problem. Validate the final problem description with practicing staff. It is important for the inter-professional team to take the time together to reflect, gather information, observe current practice, listen to clinicians, visualize how the process can be different or improved, and probe the problem description in order to develop a shared understanding of the problem.

What is the current practice?

Define the current practice as it relates to the problem. Think about current policies and procedures. Observe practices. What do you see?

How was the problem identified?

Check all the statements that apply.

What are the PICO components?

P (patient, population, problem) e.g., age, sex, setting, ethnicity, condition, disease, type of patient, or population

I (intervention) e.g., treatment, medication, education, diagnostic test, or best practice(s)

C (comparison with other interventions or current practice for foreground questions; is not applicable for background questions, which identify best practice)

O (outcomes) stated in measurable terms; may be a structure, a process, or an outcome measure based on the desired change (e.g., decrease in falls, decrease in length of stay, increase in patient satisfaction)

Initial EBP question

A starting question (usually a background question) that is often refined and adjusted as the team searches through the literature:

- *Background* questions are broad and are used when the team has little knowledge, experience, or expertise in the area of interest. Background questions are often used to identify best practices.

- *Foreground* questions are focused, with specific comparisons of two or more ideas or interventions. Foreground questions provide specific bodies of evidence related to the EBP question. Foreground questions often flow from an initial background question and literature review.

List possible search terms, databases to search, and search strategies.

Using PICO components and the initial EBP question, list search terms. Terms can be added or adjusted throughout the evidence search. Document the search terms, search strategy, and databases queried in sufficient detail for replication.

What evidence must be gathered?

Check the types of evidence the team will gather based on the PICO and initial EBP question.

Revised EBP question

Often, the question that you start with may not be the final EBP question. Background questions can be refined or changed to a foreground question based on the evidence review. Foreground questions are focused questions that include specific comparisons and produce a narrower range of evidence.

Measurement plan

Measures can be added or changed as the review of the literature is completed and the translation planning begins:

- A *measure* is an amount or a degree of something, such as number of falls with injury. Each measure must be converted to a metric, which is calculated before and after implementing the change.

- Metrics let you know whether the change was successful. They have a numerator and a denominator and are typically expressed as rates or percent. For example, a metric for the measure falls-with-injury would be the number of falls with injury (numerator) divided by 1,000 patient days (denominator). Other examples of metrics include the number of direct care RNs (numerator) on a unit divided by the total number of direct care staff (denominator); the number of medication errors divided by 1,000 orders.

Stakeholder Analysis Tool

1. Identify the key stakeholders.

- ❑ Manager or direct supervisor
- ❑ Finance department
- ❑ Vendors
- ❑ Patients and/or families; patient and family advisory committee

- ❑ Professional organizations
- ❑ Committees
- ❑ Organizational leaders
- ❑ Interdisciplinary colleagues (physicians, nutritionists, respiratory therapists, or OT/PT, for example)

- ❑ Administrators
- ❑ Other units or departments
- ❑ Others:

  _____

  _____

2. Stakeholder roles and responsibilities.

(The stakeholder roles—which include Responsibility, Consult, Approval, and Inform and their corresponding responsibilities, described here—guide completion of the table.)

Responsibility
- Completes identified tasks
- Recommending authority

Consult
- Provides input (i.e., subject matter experts)
- No decision-making authority

Approval
- Signs off on recommendations
- May veto

Inform
- Notified of progress and changes
- No input on decisions

Project tasks	Stakeholder name	Stakeholder name	Stakeholder name
	Stakeholder role	Stakeholder role	Stakeholder role

Directions for Use of the Stakeholder Analysis Tool

Purpose of the form

This form is used to identify key stakeholders. Key stakeholders are persons, groups, or departments in the organization that have an interest in, or concern about, your project and/or may assist you in securing resources to implement your action plan. Involve stakeholders early in the process to ensure their buy-in for implementation.

Because stakeholders may change at different steps of the process, we recommend that you review this form as you proceed from step to step in your action plan.

Definition

Stakeholders are "persons or groups that have a vested interest in a clinical [or nonclinical] decision and the evidence that supports that decision" (AHRQ, 2014)

Identify the key stakeholders

Identify the 5–7 key stakeholders who can most affect, or who will be most affected by, the project, actions, objectives, or change and who can influence the success of the translation work. Key stakeholders are individuals or groups who:

- Make decisions about the project
- Approve the project or aspects of the project
- Serve as subject matter experts
- Provide resources such as support, policy changes, resources, and time

Stakeholder analysis

It is helpful to consider which of the four roles each stakeholder may play in your action planning and translation work. The possible roles are:

- Responsibility

- Approval

- Consult

- Inform

Remember that one stakeholder may fill different roles, depending on the action. Completion of the Stakeholder Analysis Tool will help clarify roles and responsibilities. The descriptions of responsibilities for each role provided on the form will be helpful in this process.

References

Agency for Healthcare Research and Quality. (2014). Stakeholder Guide 2014. Retrieved from www.effectivehealthcare.ahrq.gov. AHRQ Publication No. 14-EHC010-EF. Replaces Publication No. 11-EHC069-EF

Evidence Level and Quality Guide

Evidence Levels	Quality Ratings
Level I Experimental study, randomized controlled trial (RCT) Explanatory mixed method design that includes only a level I quaNtitative study Systematic review of RCTs, with or without meta-analysis	**QuaNtitative Studies** **A High quality:** Consistent, generalizable results; sufficient sample size for the study design; adequate control; definitive conclusions; consistent recommendations based on comprehensive literature review that includes thorough reference to scientific evidence. **B Good quality:** Reasonably consistent results; sufficient sample size for the study design; some control, fairly definitive conclusions; reasonably consistent recommendations based on fairly comprehensive literature review that includes some reference to scientific evidence. **C Low quality or major flaws:** Little evidence with inconsistent results; insufficient sample size for the study design; conclusions cannot be drawn.
Level II Quasi-experimental study Explanatory mixed method design that includes only a level II quaNtitative study Systematic review of a combination of RCTs and quasi-experimental studies, or quasi-experimental studies only, with or without meta-analysis	**QuaLitative Studies** No commonly agreed-on principles exist for judging the quality of quaLitative studies. It is a subjective process based on the extent to which study data contributes to synthesis and how much information is known about the researchers' efforts to meet the appraisal criteria. *For meta-synthesis, there is preliminary agreement that quality assessments of individual studies should be made before synthesis to screen out poor-quality studies*[1]. **A/B High/Good quality** is used for single studies and meta-syntheses)[2]. The report discusses efforts to enhance or evaluate the quality of the data and the overall inquiry in sufficient detail; and it describes the specific techniques used to enhance the quality of the inquiry. Evidence of some or all of the following is found in the report: ■ **Transparency:** Describes how information was documented to justify decisions, how data were reviewed by others, and how themes and categories were formulated. ■ **Diligence:** Reads and rereads data to check interpretations; seeks opportunity to find multiple sources to corroborate evidence. ■ **Verification:** The process of checking, confirming, and ensuring methodologic coherence. ■ **Self-reflection and -scrutiny:** Being continuously aware of how a researcher's experiences, background, or prejudices might shape and bias analysis and interpretations. ■ **Participant-driven inquiry:** Participants shape the scope and breadth of questions; analysis and interpretation give voice to those who participated. ■ **Insightful interpretation:** Data and knowledge are linked in meaningful ways to relevant literature. **C Lower-quality** studies contribute little to the overall review of findings and have few, if any, of the features listed for High/Good quality.
Level III Nonexperimental study Systematic review of a combination of RCTs, quasi-experimental and nonexperimental studies, or nonexperimental studies only, with or without meta-analysis Exploratory, convergent, or multiphasic mixed methods studies Explanatory mixed method design that includes only a level III quaNtitative study QuaLitative study Meta-synthesis	

Evidence Levels	Quality Ratings
Level IV Opinion of respected authorities and/or nationally recognized expert committees or consensus panels based on scientific evidence Includes: ■ Clinical practice guidelines ■ Consensus panels/position statements	**A** <u>High quality:</u> Material officially sponsored by a professional, public, or private organization or a government agency; documentation of a systematic literature search strategy; consistent results with sufficient numbers of well-designed studies; criteria-based evaluation of overall scientific strength and quality of included studies and definitive conclusions; national expertise clearly evident; developed or revised within the past five years **B** <u>Good quality:</u> Material officially sponsored by a professional, public, or private organization or a government agency; reasonably thorough and appropriate systematic literature search strategy; reasonably consistent results, sufficient numbers of well-designed studies; evaluation of strengths and limitations of included studies with fairly definitive conclusions; national expertise clearly evident; developed or revised within the past five years **C** <u>Low quality or major flaws:</u> Material not sponsored by an official organization or agency; undefined, poorly defined, or limited literature search strategy; no evaluation of strengths and limitations of included studies, insufficient evidence with inconsistent results, conclusions cannot be drawn; not revised within the past five years
Level V Based on experiential and nonresearch evidence Includes: ■ Integrative reviews ■ Literature reviews ■ Quality improvement, program, or financial evaluation ■ Case reports ■ Opinion of nationally recognized expert(s) based on experiential evidence	**Organizational Experience** (quality improvement, program or financial evaluation) **A** <u>High quality:</u> Clear aims and objectives; consistent results across multiple settings; formal quality improvement, financial, or program evaluation methods used; definitive conclusions; consistent recommendations with thorough reference to scientific evidence **B** <u>Good quality:</u> Clear aims and objectives; consistent results in a single setting; formal quality improvement, financial, or program evaluation methods used; reasonably consistent recommendations with some reference to scientific evidence **C** <u>Low quality or major flaws:</u> Unclear or missing aims and objectives; inconsistent results; poorly defined quality improvement, financial, or program evaluation methods; recommendations cannot be made **Integrative Review, Literature Review, Expert Opinion, Case Report, Community Standard, Clinician Experience, Consumer Preference** **A** <u>High quality:</u> Expertise is clearly evident; draws definitive conclusions; provides scientific rationale; thought leader(s) in the field **B** <u>Good quality:</u> Expertise appears to be credible; draws fairly definitive conclusions; provides logical argument for opinions **C** <u>Low quality or major flaws:</u> Expertise is not discernable or is dubious; conclusions cannot be drawn

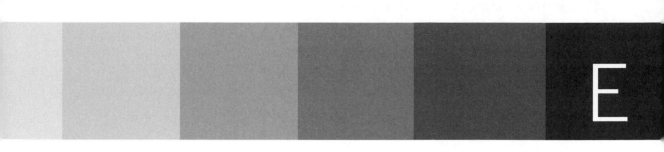

Research Evidence
Appraisal Tool

Evidence level and quality rating:	_____
Article title:	Number:
Author(s):	Publication date:
Journal:	

Setting:	Sample (composition and size):	
Does this evidence address my EBP question?	❏ Yes	❏ No Do not proceed with appraisal of this evidence.

Is this study:

- **QuaNtitative** (collection, analysis, and reporting of numerical data)

  Measurable data (how many; how much; or how often) used to formulate facts, uncover patterns in research, and generalize results from a larger sample population; provides observed effects of a program, problem, or condition, measured precisely, rather than through researcher interpretation of data. Common methods are surveys, face-to-face structured interviews, observations, and reviews of records or documents. Statistical tests are used in data analysis.

  Go to **Section I: QuaNtitative**

- **QuaLitative** (collection, analysis, and reporting of narrative data)

  Rich narrative documents are used for uncovering themes; describes a problem or condition from the point of view of those experiencing it. Common methods are focus groups, individual interviews (unstructured or semistructured), and participation/observations. Sample sizes are small and are determined when data saturation is achieved. Data saturation is reached when the researcher identifies that no new themes emerge and redundancy is occurring. Synthesis is used in data analysis. Often a starting point for studies when little research exists; may use results to design empirical studies. The researcher describes, analyzes, and interprets reports, descriptions, and observations from participants.

  Go to **Section II: QuaLitative**

- Mixed methods (results reported both numerically and narratively)

  Both quaNtitative and quaLitative methods are used in the study design. Using both approaches, in combination, provides a better understanding of research problems than using either approach alone. Sample sizes vary based on methods used. Data collection involves collecting and analyzing both quaNtitative and quaLitative data in a single study or series of studies. Interpretation is continual and can influence stages in the research process.

  Go to **Section I** for QuaNtitative components and **Section II** for QuaLitative components

Section I: QuaNtitative

Level of Evidence (Study Design)

| A. Is this a report of a single research study? | | ❑ Yes | ❑ No
Go to B. |
|---|---|---|---|
| 1. Was there manipulation of an independent variable? | | ❑ Yes | ❑ No |
| 2. Was there a control group? | | ❑ Yes | ❑ No |
| 3. Were study participants randomly assigned to the intervention and control groups? | | ❑ Yes | ❑ No |
| If Yes to questions 1, 2, and 3, this is a randomized controlled trial (RCT) or experimental study. | ❑ LEVEL I | | |
| If Yes to questions 1 and 2 and No to question 3, *or* Yes to question 1 and No to questions 2 and 3, this is quasi-experimental (some degree of investigator control, some manipulation of an independent variable, lacks random assignment to groups, and may have a control group). | ❑ LEVEL II | | |
| If No to questions 1, 2, and 3, this is nonexperimental (no manipulation of independent variable; can be descriptive, comparative, or correlational; often uses secondary data). | ❑ LEVEL III | | |
| Study Findings That Help Answer the EBP Question | | | |

Complete the Appraisal of QuaNtitative Research Studies section.

B. Is this a summary of multiple sources of research evidence?		❏ Yes Continue	❏ No Go to Appendix F
1. Does it employ a comprehensive search strategy and rigorous appraisal method? If this study includes research, nonresearch, and experiential evidence, it is an integrative review. See Appendix F.		❏ Yes	❏ No Go to Appendix F

2. For systematic reviews and systematic reviews with meta-analysis (see descriptions below):
 	
   a. Are all studies included RCTs?
 	
   b. Are the studies a combination of RCTs and quasi-experimental, or quasi-experimental only?
 	
   c. Are the studies a combination of RCTs, quasi-experimental, and nonexperimental, or non-experimental only?
 	
A <u>systematic review</u> employs a search strategy and a rigorous appraisal method, but does not generate an effect size.
 	
A <u>meta-analysis</u>, or systematic review with meta-analysis, combines and analyzes results from studies to generate a new statistic: the effect size.
	❏ Level I
	
	❏ Level II
	
	❏ Level III		

Study Findings That Help Answer the EBP Question			
Complete the Appraisal of Systematic Review (With or Without a Meta-Analysis) section.			

Appraisal of QuaNtitative Research Studies			
Does the researcher identify what is known and not known about the problem and how the study will address any gaps in knowledge?	❏ Yes	❏ No	
Was the purpose of the study clearly presented?	❏ Yes	❏ No	
Was the literature review current (most sources within the past five years or a seminal study)?	❏ Yes	❏ No	
Was sample size sufficient based on study design and rationale?	❏ Yes	❏ No	
If there is a control group: ▪ Were the characteristics and/or demographics similar in both the control and intervention groups?	❏ Yes	❏ No	❏ N/A
▪ If multiple settings were used, were the settings similar?	❏ Yes	❏ No	❏ N/A
▪ Were all groups equally treated except for the intervention group(s)?	❏ Yes	❏ No	❏ N/A
Are data collection methods described clearly?	❏ Yes	❏ No	
Were the instruments reliable (Cronbach's α [alpha] > 0.70)?	❏ Yes	❏ No	❏ N/A
Was instrument validity discussed?	❏ Yes	❏ No	❏ N/A
If surveys or questionnaires were used, was the response rate $\geq$ 25%?	❏ Yes	❏ No	❏ N/A
Were the results presented clearly?	❏ Yes	❏ No	
If tables were presented, was the narrative consistent with the table content?	❏ Yes	❏ No	❏ N/A
Were study limitations identified and addressed?	❏ Yes	❏ No	
Were conclusions based on results?	❏ Yes	❏ No	
Go to Quality Rating for QuaNtitative Studies section			
Appraisal of Systematic Review (With or Without Meta-Analysis)			
Were the variables of interest clearly identified?	❏ Yes	❏ No	
Was the search comprehensive and reproducible? ▪ Key search terms stated	❏ Yes	❏ No	
▪ Multiple databases searched and identified	❏ Yes	❏ No	
▪ Inclusion and exclusion criteria stated	❏ Yes	❏ No	
Was there a flow diagram that included the number of studies eliminated at each level of review?	❏ Yes	❏ No	

Were details of included studies presented (design, sample, methods, results, outcomes, strengths, and limitations?	❏ Yes	❏ No
Were methods for appraising the strength of evidence (level and quality) described?	❏ Yes	❏ No
Were conclusions based on results?	❏ Yes	❏ No
▪ Results were interpreted.	❏ Yes	❏ No
▪ Conclusions flowed logically from the interpretation and systematic review question.	❏ Yes	❏ No
Did the systematic review include a section addressing limitations *and* how they were addressed?	❏ Yes	❏ No

Quality Rating for QuaNtitative Studies

Complete quality rating for quaNtitative studies section.

Circle the appropriate quality rating below

A High quality: Consistent, generalizable results; sufficient sample size for the study design; adequate control; definitive conclusions; consistent recommendations based on comprehensive literature review that includes thorough reference to scientific evidence.

B Good quality: Reasonably consistent results; sufficient sample size for the study design; some control, and fairly definitive conclusions; reasonably consistent recommendations based on fairly comprehensive literature review that includes some reference to scientific evidence.

C Low quality or major flaws: Little evidence with inconsistent results; insufficient sample size for the study design; conclusions cannot be drawn.

Section II: QuaLitative

Level of Evidence (Study Design)

A. Is this a report of a single quaLitative research study?	❏ Yes Level III	❏ No Go to Section II. B
Study Findings That Help Answer the EBP Question		

Complete the Appraisal of Single QuaLitative Research Study section.

Appraisal of a Single QuaLitative Research Study

Was there a clearly identifiable and articulated:		
▪ Purpose?	❑ Yes	❑ No
▪ Research question?	❑ Yes	❑ No
▪ Justification for method(s) used?	❑ Yes	❑ No
▪ Phenomenon that is the focus of the research?	❑ Yes	❑ No
Were study sample participants representative?	❑ Yes	❑ No
Did they have knowledge of or experience with the research area?	❑ Yes	❑ No
Were participant characteristics described?	❑ Yes	❑ No
Was sampling adequate, as evidenced by achieving saturation of data?	❑ Yes	❑ No
Data analysis: ▪ Was a verification process used in every step by checking and confirming with participants the trustworthiness of analysis and interpretation?	❑ Yes	❑ No
▪ Was there a description of how data were analyzed (i.e., method), by computer or manually?	❑ Yes	❑ No
Do findings support the narrative data (quotes)?	❑ Yes	❑ No
Do findings flow from research question to data collected to analysis undertaken?	❑ Yes	❑ No
Are conclusions clearly explained?	❑ Yes	❑ No
Go to Quality Rating for QuaLitative Studies section.		
B. For summaries of multiple quaLitative research studies (meta-synthesis), was a comprehensive search strategy and rigorous appraisal method used?	❑ Yes Level III	❑ No Go to Appendix F.

Study Findings That Help Answer the EBP Question

Complete the Appraisal of Meta-Synthesis Studies section.

Appraisal of Meta-Synthesis Studies		
Were the search strategy and criteria for selecting primary studies clearly defined?	❑ Yes	❑ No
Were findings appropriate and convincing?	❑ Yes	❑ No
Was a description of methods used to:		
▪ Compare findings from each study?	❑ Yes	❑ No
▪ Interpret data?	❑ Yes	❑ No
Did synthesis reflect:		
▪ New insights?	❑ Yes	❑ No
▪ Discovery of essential features of phenomena?	❑ Yes	❑ No
▪ A fuller understanding of the phenomena?	❑ Yes	❑ No
Was sufficient data presented to support the interpretations?	❑ Yes	❑ No
Complete Quality Rating for QuaLitative Studies section.		
Quality Rating for QuaLitative Studies		

Circle the appropriate quality rating below

No commonly agreed-on principles exist for judging the quality of quaLitative studies. It is a subjective process based on the extent to which study data contributes to synthesis and how much information is known about the researchers' efforts to meet the appraisal criteria.

For meta-synthesis, there is preliminary agreement that quality assessments should be made before synthesis to screen out poor-quality studies[1].

A/B   High/Good quality is used for single studies and meta-syntheses)[2].

The report discusses efforts to enhance or evaluate the quality of the data and the overall inquiry in sufficient detail; and it describes the specific techniques used to enhance the quality of the inquiry. Evidence of some or all of the following is found in the report:

- **Transparency:** Describes how information was documented to justify decisions, how data were reviewed by others, and how themes and categories were formulated.
- **Diligence:** Reads and rereads data to check interpretations; seeks opportunity to find multiple sources to corroborate evidence.
- **Verification:** The process of checking, confirming, and ensuring methodologic coherence.
- **Self-reflection and self-scrutiny:** Being continuously aware of how a researcher's experiences, background, or prejudices might shape and bias analysis and interpretations.
- **Participant-driven inquiry:** Participants shape the scope and breadth of questions; analysis and interpretation give voice to those who participated.
- **Insightful interpretation:** Data and knowledge are linked in meaningful ways to relevant literature.

C   **Lower-quality** studies contribute little to the overall review of findings and have few, if any, of the features listed for High/Good quality.

Section III: Mixed Methods

Level of Evidence (Study Design)

You will need to appraise both the quaNtitative and quaLitative parts of the study independently, before appraising the study in its entirety.		
1. Evaluate the quaNtitative portion of the study using Section I. Insert here the level of evidence and overall quality for this part:	Level __	Quality __
2. Evaluate the quaLitative part of the study using Section II. Insert here the level of evidence and overall quality for this part:	Level __	Quality __
3. To determine the level of evidence, circle the appropriate study design: (a) **Explanatory** sequential designs collect quaNtitative data first, followed by the quaLitative data; and their purpose is to explain quaNtitative results using quaLitative findings. The level is determined based on the level of the quaNtitative part. (b) **Exploratory** sequential designs collect quaLitative data first, followed by the quaNtitative data; and their purpose is to explain quaLitative findings using the quaNtitative results. The level is determined based on the level of the quaLitative part, and it is always Level III. (c) **Convergent** parallel designs collect the quaLitative and quaNtitative data concurrently for the purpose of providing a more complete understanding of a phenomenon by merging both datasets. These designs are Level III. (d) **Multiphasic** designs collect quaLitative and quaNtitative data over more than one phase, with each phase informing the next phase. These designs are Level III.		

Study Findings That Help Answer the EBP Question

Use the Appraisal of Mixed Methods Studies section.

Appraisal of Mixed Methods Studies[3]			
Was the mixed-methods research design relevant to address the quaNtitative and quaLitative research questions (or objectives)?	❏ Yes	❏ No	❏ N/A
Was the research design relevant to address the quaNtitative and quaLitative aspects of the mixed-methods question (or objective)?	❏ Yes	❏ No	❏ N/A
For convergent parallel designs, was the integration of quaNtitative and quaLitative data (or results) relevant to address the research question or objective?	❏ Yes	❏ No	❏ N/A
For convergent parallel designs, were the limitations associated with the integration (for example, the divergence of quaLitative and quaNtitative data or results) sufficiently addressed?	❏ Yes	❏ No	❏ N/A

Quality Rating for Mixed-Methods Studies

Circle the appropriate quality rating below

A High quality: Contains high-quality quaNtitative and quaLitative study components; highly relevant study design; relevant integration of data or results; and careful consideration of the limitations of the chosen approach.

B Good quality: Contains good-quality quaNtitative and quaLitative study components; relevant study design; moderately relevant integration of data or results; and some discussion of limitations of integration.

C Low quality or major flaws: Contains low quality quaNtitative and quaLitative study components; study design not relevant to research questions or objectives; poorly integrated data or results; and no consideration of limits of integration.

1 https://www.york.ac.uk/crd/SysRev/!SSL!/WebHelp/6_4_ASSESSMENT_OF_QUALITATIVE_RESEARCH.htm

2 Adapted from Polit & Beck (2017).

3 National Collaborating Centre for Methods and Tools. (2015). Appraising Qualitative, Quantitative, and Mixed Methods Studies included in Mixed Studies Reviews: The MMAT. Hamilton, ON: McMaster University. (Updated 20 July, 2015) Retrieved from http://www.nccmt.ca/resources/search/232

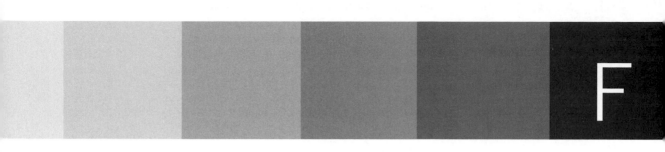

Nonresearch Evidence
Appraisal Tool

Evidence level and quality rating:	_____	
Article title:	Number:	
Author(s):	Publication date:	
Journal:		
Setting:	Sample (composition and size):	
Does this evidence address my EBP question?	❑ Yes	❑ No Do not proceed with appraisal of this evidence.

❑ **Clinical Practice Guidelines LEVEL IV** **Systematically developed recommendations from nationally recognized experts based on research evidence or expert consensus panel** ❑ **Consensus or Position Statement LEVEL IV** **Systematically developed recommendations, based on research and nationally recognized expert opinion, that guide members of a professional organization in decision-making for an issue of concern**		
▪ Are the types of evidence included identified?	❑ Yes	❑ No
▪ Were appropriate stakeholders involved in the development of recommendations?	❑ Yes	❑ No
▪ Are groups to which recommendations apply and do not apply clearly stated?	❑ Yes	❑ No
▪ Have potential biases been eliminated?	❑ Yes	❑ No
▪ Does each recommendation have an identified level of evidence stated?	❑ Yes	❑ No
▪ Are recommendations clear?	❑ Yes	❑ No
Complete the corresponding quality rating section.		

❏ **Literature review LEVEL V**
Summary of selected published literature including scientific and nonscientific such as reports of organizational experience and opinions of experts

❏ **Integrative review LEVEL V**
Summary of research evidence and theoretical literature; analyzes, compares themes, notes gaps in the selected literature

■ Is subject matter to be reviewed clearly stated?	❏ Yes	❏ No
■ Is literature relevant and up-to-date (most sources are within the past five years or classic)?	❏ Yes	❏ No
■ Of the literature reviewed, is there a meaningful analysis of the conclusions across the articles included in the review?	❏ Yes	❏ No
■ Are gaps in the literature identified?	❏ Yes	❏ No
■ Are recommendations made for future practice or study?	❏ Yes	❏ No

Complete the corresponding quality rating.

❏ **Expert opinion LEVEL V**
Opinion of one or more individuals based on clinical expertise

■ Has the individual published or presented on the topic?	❏ Yes	❏ No
■ Is the author's opinion based on scientific evidence?	❏ Yes	❏ No
■ Is the author's opinion clearly stated?	❏ Yes	❏ No
■ Are potential biases acknowledged?	❏ Yes	❏ No

Complete the corresponding quality rating.

Organizational Experience

❏ **Quality improvement LEVEL V**
Cyclical method to examine workflows, processes, or systems with a specific organization

❏ **Financial evaluation LEVEL V**
Economic evaluation that applies analytic techniques to identify, measure, and compare the cost and outcomes of two or more alternative programs or interventions

❏ **Program evaluation LEVEL V**
Systematic assessment of the processes and/or outcomes of a program; can involve both quaNtitative and quaLitative methods

Setting	Sample Composition/Size		
■ Was the aim of the project clearly stated?	❑ Yes	❑ No	
■ Was the method fully described?	❑ Yes	❑ No	
■ Were process or outcome measures identified?	❑ Yes	❑ No	
■ Were results fully described?	❑ Yes	❑ No	
■ Was interpretation clear and appropriate?	❑ Yes	❑ No	
■ Are components of cost/benefit or cost effectiveness analysis described?	❑ Yes	❑ No	❑ N/A
Complete the corresponding quality rating.			
❑ Case report LEVEL V **In-depth look at a person or group or another social unit**			
■ Is the purpose of the case report clearly stated?	❑ Yes	❑ No	
■ Is the case report clearly presented?	❑ Yes	❑ No	
■ Are the findings of the case report supported by relevant theory or research?	❑ Yes	❑ No	
■ Are the recommendations clearly stated and linked to the findings?	❑ Yes	❑ No	
Complete the corresponding quality rating.			
Community standard, clinician experience, or consumer preference LEVEL V **❑ Community standard:** Current practice for comparable settings in the community **❑ Clinician experience:** Knowledge gained through practice experience **❑ Consumer preference:** Knowledge gained through life experience			
Information Source(s)	**Number of Sources**		
■ Source of information has credible experience.	❑ Yes	❑ No	
■ Opinions are clearly stated.	❑ Yes	❑ No	❑ N/A
■ Evidence obtained is consistent.	❑ Yes	❑ No	❑ N/A
Findings That Help You Answer the EBP Question			

Quality Rating for Clinical Practice Guidelines, Consensus, or Position Statements (Level IV)

A. High quality

Material officially sponsored by a professional, public, or private organization or a government agency; documentation of a systematic literature search strategy; consistent results with sufficient numbers of well-designed studies; criteria-based evaluation of overall scientific strength and quality of included studies and definitive conclusions; national expertise clearly evident; developed or revised within the past five years.

B. Good quality

Material officially sponsored by a professional, public, or private organization or a government agency; reasonably thorough and appropriate systematic literature search strategy; reasonably consistent results, sufficient numbers of well-designed studies; evaluation of strengths and limitations of included studies with fairly definitive conclusions; national expertise clearly evident; developed or revised within the past five years.

C. Low quality or major flaw

Material not sponsored by an official organization or agency; undefined, poorly defined, or limited literature search strategy; no evaluation of strengths and limitations of included studies; insufficient evidence with inconsistent results; conclusions cannot be drawn; not revised within the past five years.

Quality Rating for Organizational Experience (Level V)

A. High quality

Clear aims and objectives; consistent results across multiple settings; formal quality improvement or financial evaluation methods used; definitive conclusions; consistent recommendations with thorough reference to scientific evidence.

B. Good quality

Clear aims and objectives; formal quality improvement or financial evaluation methods used; consistent results in a single setting; reasonably consistent recommendations with some reference to scientific evidence.

C. Low quality or major flaws

Unclear or missing aims and objectives; inconsistent results; poorly defined quality; improvement/financial analysis method; recommendations cannot be made.

Quality Rating for Case Report, Integrative Review, Literature Review, Expert Opinion, Community Standard, Clinician Experience, Consumer Preference (Level V)

A. High quality

Expertise is clearly evident, draws definitive conclusions, and provides scientific rationale; thought leader in the field.

B. Good quality

Expertise appears to be credible, draws fairly definitive conclusions, and provides logical argument for opinions.

C. Low quality or major flaws

Expertise is not discernable or is dubious; conclusions cannot be drawn.

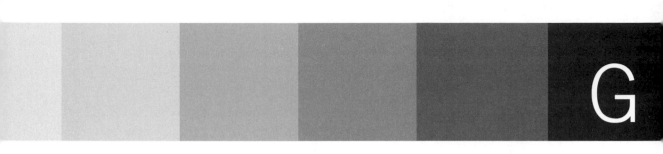

Individual Evidence
Summary Tool

EBP Question:

Date:

Article Number	Author and Date	Evidence Type	Sample, Sample Size, Setting	Findings That Help Answer the EBP Question	Observable Measures	Limitations	Evidence Level, Quality
			☐ N/A				
			☐ N/A				
			☐ N/A				
			☐ N/A				
			☐ N/A				
			☐ N/A				
			☐ N/A				

Attach a reference list with full citations of articles reviewed for this EBP question.

Directions for Use of the Individual Evidence Summary Tool

Purpose

This form is used to document the results of evidence appraisal in preparation for evidence synthesis. The form provides the EBP team with documentation of the sources of evidence used, the year the evidence was published or otherwise communicated, the information gathered from each evidence source that helps the team answer the EBP question, and the level and quality of each source of evidence.

Article Number

Assign a number to each reviewed source of evidence. This organizes the individual evidence summary and provides an easy way to reference articles.

Author and Date

Indicate the last name of the first author or the evidence source and the publication/communication date. List both author/evidence source and date.

Evidence Type

Indicate the type of evidence reviewed (for example: RCT, meta-analysis, mixed methods, quaLitative, systematic review, case study, narrative literature review).

Sample, Sample Size, and Setting

Provide a quick view of the population, number of participants, and study location.

Findings That Help Answer the EBP Question

Although the reviewer may find many points of interest, list only findings that directly apply to the EBP question.

Observable Measures

QuaNtitative measures or variables are used to answer a research question, test a hypothesis, describe characteristics, or determine the effect, impact, or influence. QuaLitative evidence uses cases, context, opinions, experiences, and thoughts to represent the phenomenon of study.

Limitations

Include information that may or may not be within the text of the article regarding drawbacks of the piece of evidence. The evidence may list limitations, or it may be evident to you, as you review the evidence, that an important point is missed or the sample does not apply to the population of interest.

Evidence Level and Quality

Using information from the individual appraisal tools, transfer the evidence level and quality rating into this column.

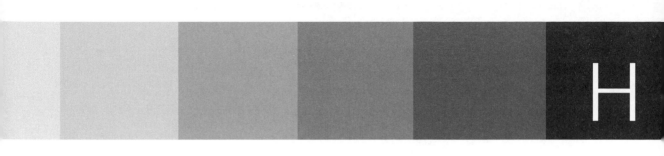

H

Synthesis Process and Recommendations Tool

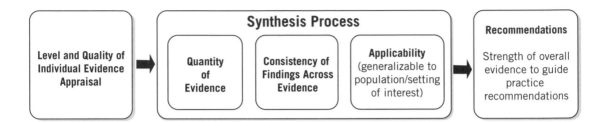

Key Points:

- Evidence synthesis is best done through group discussion. All team members share their perspectives, and the team uses critical thinking to arrive at a judgment based on consensus during the synthesis process. The synthesis process involves both subjective and objective reasoning by the full EBP team.

  Through reasoning, the team:

  - Reviews the quality appraisal of the individual pieces of evidence

  - Assesses and assimilates consistencies in findings

  - Evaluates the meaning and relevance of the findings

  - Merges findings that may either enhance the team's knowledge or generate new insights, perspectives, and understandings

  - Highlights inconsistencies in findings

  - Makes recommendations based on the synthesis process.

- When evidence includes multiple studies of Level I and Level II evidence, there is a similar population or setting of interest, and there is consistency across findings, EBP teams can have greater confidence in recommending a practice change. However, with a majority of Level II and Level III evidence, the team should proceed cautiously in making practice changes. In this instance, recommendation(s) typically include completing a pilot before deciding to implement a full-scale change.

- Generally, practice changes are not made on Level IV or Level V evidence alone. Nonetheless, teams have a variety of options for actions that include, but are not limited to: creating awareness campaigns, conducting informational and educational updates, monitoring evidence sources for new information, and designing research studies.

- The quality rating (see Appendix D) is used to appraise both individual quality of evidence and overall quality of evidence.

EBP Question:

Category (Level Type)	Total Number of Sources/ Level	Overall Quality Rating	Synthesis of Findings Evidence That Answers the EBP Question
Level I ■ Experimental study ■ Randomized controlled trial (RCT) ■ Systematic review of RCTs with or without meta-analysis ■ Explanatory mixed method design that includes only a Level I quaNtitative study			
Level II ■ Quasi-experimental studies ■ Systematic review of a combination of RCTs and quasi-experimental studies, or quasi-experimental studies only, with or without meta-analysis ■ Explanatory mixed method design that includes only a Level II quaNtitative study			

continues

Category (Level Type)	Total Number of Sources/ Level	Overall Quality Rating	Synthesis of Findings Evidence That Answers the EBP Question
Level III ■ Nonexperimental study ■ Systematic review of a combination of RCTs, quasi-experimental and nonexperimental studies, or nonexperimental studies only, with or without meta-analysis ■ QuaLitative study or meta-synthesis ■ Exploratory, convergent, or multiphasic mixed-methods studies ■ Explanatory mixed method design that includes only a level III QuaNtitative study			
Level IV ■ Opinions of respected authorities and/or reports of nationally recognized expert committees or consensus panels based on scientific evidence			
Level V ■ Evidence obtained from literature or integrative reviews, quality improvement, program evaluation, financial evaluation, or case reports ■ Opinion of nationally recognized expert(s) based on experiential evidence			

Based on your synthesis, which of the following four pathways to translation represents the overall strength of the evidence?

❏   Strong, compelling evidence, consistent results: Solid indication for a practice change is indicated.

❏   Good and consistent evidence: Consider pilot of change or further investigation.

❏   Good but conflicting evidence: No indication for practice change; consider further investigation for new evidence or develop a research study.

❏   Little or no evidence: No indication for practice change; consider further investigation for new evidence, develop a research study, or discontinue project.

If you selected either the first option or the second option, continue. If not, *STOP*—translation is not indicated.

Recommendations based on evidence synthesis and selected translation pathway

Consider the following as you examine *fit*:

Are the recommendations:

- Compatible with the unit/departmental/organizational cultural values or norms?

- Consistent with unit/departmental/organizational assumptions, structures, attitudes, beliefs, and/or practices?

- Consistent with the unit/departmental/organizational priorities?

Consider the following questions as you examine *feasibility*:

- Can we do what they did in our work environment?
- Are the following supports available?
    - Resources
    - Funding
    - Approval from administration and clinical leaders
    - Stakeholder support
- Is it likely that the recommendations can be implemented within the unit/department/organization?

Directions for Use of This Form

Purpose of form

Use this form to compile the results of the individual evidence appraisal to answer the EBP question. The pertinent findings for each level of evidence are synthesized, and a quality rating is assigned to each level.

Total number of sources per level

Record the number of sources of evidence for each level.

Overall quality rating

Summarize the overall quality of evidence for each level. Use Appendix D to rate the quality of evidence.

Synthesis of findings: evidence that answers the EBP question

- Include only findings from evidence of A or B quality.

- Include only statements that directly answer the EBP question.

- Summarize findings within each level of evidence.

- Record article number(s) from individual evidence summary in parentheses next to each statement so that the source of the finding is easy to identify.

Develop recommendations based on evidence synthesis and the selected translation pathway

Review the synthesis of findings and determine which of the following four pathways to translation represents the overall strength of the evidence:

- Strong, compelling evidence, consistent results: Solid indication for a practice change is indicated.

- Good and consistent evidence: Consider pilot of change or further investigation.

- Good but conflicting evidence: No indication for practice change; consider further investigation for new evidence or develop a research study.

- Little or no evidence: No indication for practice change; consider further investigation for new evidence, develop a research study, or discontinue the project.

Fit and feasibility

Even when evidence is strong and of high quality, it may not be appropriate to implement a change in practice. It is crucial to examine feasibility that considers the resources available, the readiness for change, and the balance between risk and benefit. *Fit* refers to the compatibility of the proposed change with the organization's mission, goals, objectives, and priorities. A change that does not fit within the organizational priorities will be less likely to receive leadership and financial support, making success difficult. Implementing processes with a low likelihood of success wastes valuable time and resources on efforts that produce negligible benefits.

Action Planning Tool

1. Complete the following activities to ensure successful translation:

❑ Secure a project leader.

❑ Consider whether translation activities require different or additional members.

❑ Identify critical milestones and related tasks.

❑ Identify change champions.

❑ Schedule time to complete milestones.

❑ Identify observable pre- or post-measures.

2. Identify barriers to the success of the change, and then identify strengths that can be leveraged to overcome barriers.

Barriers	Resources or Strengths	Plan to Overcome Barriers by Leveraging Strengths as Appropriate

3. Consider whether or how this change will affect the following:

❑ Electronic health record

❑ Workflow

❑ Policies and/or procedures

4. Confirm support and/or availability of funds to cover expenses. (Check all that apply.)

❑ Personnel costs

❑ Supplies/equipment

❑ Technology

❑ Photocopying

❑ Education or further training

❑ Content or external experts

❑ Dissemination costs (conference costs, travel)

❑ Other: _____

5. Identify critical milestones and related tasks:				
	(Insert Milestone 1)	*(Insert Milestone 2)*	*(Insert Milestone 3)*	*(Insert Milestone 4)*
Tasks	*(Insert task)*			

Directions for Use of the Action Planning Tool

Purpose of form

This form is used to guide you as you create an action plan.

Activities to ensure successful translation

These are all activities that must be completed as you plan the change. Consider pre- and post-observable measures that can be used to determine whether the change was successful. In addition, identifying critical milestones allows the team to see whether they are on track to accomplish the goals.

Identify strengths/resources and barriers to the success of the change

This analysis allows teams to identify barriers to implementation and potentially mitigate them using inherent strengths and resources. You may find specific challenges that will likely impact the ability to deliver on the action plan. Though these obstacles can get in the way, knowing about them up front is helpful so that you can engage support and create a plan to address them.

Consider whether or how the change will impact workflows and processes

Be mindful of the impact of the change downstream. For example, will changes need to be made to the electronic medical record to accommodate the change, or will this change impact the workflow of any other staff who have not been considered?

Confirm support and/or availability of funds to cover expenses

Use this as a guide to prompt thoughtfulness about financial obligations that may be a part of the rollout.

Identify critical milestones and related tasks

Consider all the categories of work (milestones) necessary to implement this change. What tasks must be accomplished first for each milestone in order to move forward? When must they be completed to stay on track? For example, if a milestone is to implement a protocol, list all tasks to accomplish it.

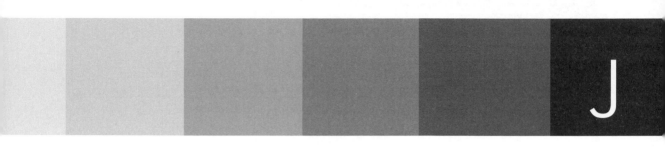

Dissemination Tool

1. Think about the project findings and practice change initiative. What is the most important information you need to convey?

2. Align key messages with audiences.

Audience	Key Message	Communication Method
Interdisciplinary stakeholders		
Organizational leadership		
Departmental leadership		
Frontline staff		
External community (publications, posters, and presentations)		

3. Review examples below to identify appropriate communication methods.

- ❏ Written publication
- ❏ External conference
- ❏ Poster presentation
- ❏ Internal meeting / inservice
- ❏ Audio / video content

- ❏ Online program
- ❏ Podium presentation
- ❏ Social media blast
- ❏ Others: _____

Directions for Use of the Dissemination Tool

Purpose

This form is useful at various points in the EBP project process. It is usually completed toward the end of the project, when findings are known and efforts have produced a product, tool, program, or policy.

Align key message with audience

Think about the project findings. What has the project effort accomplished? What products, policy changes, or outcomes can you report? Identify the end users—who is your audience? Your audience may be individuals, organizations, or networks who might have an interest in the project outcomes.

Communication method

This is the communication plan, and it can occur on many levels. Think about reaching the varied audiences using a multitude of methods. These can include, but are not limited to, written text, audio / visual content, online programs, and poster presentations.

Index

B

D

E

I

J

Q

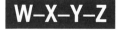